Why Does Grandma Kun Barefoot?

The Key to Fun Movement and Good Balance

Laura Blodgett

Daily Improvisations Press
in cooperation with
Fun Fitness After 50
2016

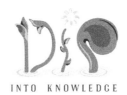

INTO KNOWLEDGE

Front cover sketch by
Katerina Zagore
worldforlove on fiverr.com

illustrations courtesy of Clinton Voris
ArtisticBusinessConsulting.weebly.com

To my husband, Greg, who accidentally introduced me to barefoot running.

To my several grown children,
who have shared the barefoot running journey with me.

To my many friends at the
Barefoot Runners Society,
who humbly share the wisdom of experience.

All the information offered herein is for guidelines and suggestions only. Each person is responsible for making careful decisions about his or her own barefoot adventures.

Contents

Foreward
by "Barefoot Rick" Roeber

I love barefoot running. As a matter of fact, I love going barefoot as much as possible. So, when Laura Blodgett asked me to write a forward to her new book *Why Does Grandma Run Barefoot?: The Key to Fun Movement and Good Balance*, I was first honored to comment on her new work, but also to help set the record straight about being barefoot as it is expressed through barefoot running.

For those of us who have lived barefoot for a good portion of our lives, barefoot running seemed like the most natural evolution from shod running. Most of us were taught by other runners and the shoe companies that we needed to conform to societal norms and understand they knew more than our primal fathers regarding our desire to go sans shoes. However, once we took off the shoes and tried barefoot running, it became "unpainfully" clear that we had hit pay dirt. Most if not all of us would never be the same runner after experiencing the joy of barefoot running.

Like Laura, my epiphany came on my first barefoot run. Similarly, I overdid it and yet loved the experience. We both knew that we were on to something. I often kid folks and tell them I was a natural for barefoot running—either too much hillbilly in my soul or closer to the Neanderthal gene pool than others! Whatever the reason, I relate with Laura's experience of encountering an inner awareness that this is the way I would run whenever possible for the rest of my life.

I have written several reviews and/or forewords for other barefoot running books. However, I was struck by how poignantly Laura explains why she runs barefoot. The first few chapters are wholly devoted to laying out a case in a rather substantial manner. What makes her defense so effective compared to some others I have read and commented on is her anecdotal testimonials that allow the reader to commiserate with her point of view. Some writers might tend to condescend to say, "By golly, it's my way or the highway!" regarding living a barefoot lifestyle. Laura's touch of humility and genuineness allows the reader to respect her even if they might not totally agree.

The "how" of barefoot running is essential once someone embraces the "why?" In this regard, Laura effectively lays out reasonable assumptions regarding barefoot running mechanics. One section I appreciated was her section on running in extreme weather. I have successfully run in snow and temps in the teens Fahrenheit and I think she gives great advice on keeping the core warm and allowing the parts that are exercising (e.g., our feet) to warm up accordingly. There is practical advice in the following: "Good circulation helps to keep the feet and the whole body warm in winter, as well as dissipate heat in summer." There are plenty of other nuggets of wisdom such as this that will help a barefoot runner be successful in any weather.

As someone who has run over 100 marathons (with most of those barefoot), I understand what is needed for successful barefoot running. Having run nearly 27,000 barefoot miles in the past 13 years qualifies me to speak with some authority on the subject. You will not regret reading this small volume, and at least giving barefoot running a try if you have never considered it. Laura weaves candidness and humor throughout these pages and allows the reader to view her experience and expertise through the eyes of someone who loves life. She bares her soul in such a way that you can't but respect her and the joy she has encountered during her barefoot journey. To one degree or another, barefooting is for everyone. You may not run barefoot marathons, or live barefoot after reading this book. However, you will find your life changed for the better if you glean just some of the wisdom in the small book and put it into practice. May you encounter joy, spirituality, and healthier living as you embrace these truths!

"Barefoot Rick" Roeber
http://barefootrunner.org

Chapter One

Who Runs Barefoot, Anyway?

What Do You Think a Barefoot Runner Looks Like?

What do you envision a barefoot runner looks like? A mental hospital escapee? Maybe someone who seems impervious to the elements of nature, able to jump in cold lakes? Possibly a devoted spiritual hermit who lives in a forest hovel and eschews modern conveniences? You probably don't picture an

average and ordinary,
over 50 year old grandmother,
married to her engineer for 34 years and
mother of their 7 grown children,
grandmother of 8,
who likes to be comfortable.

But that would be me, and I run barefoot.

I really do run. Admittedly, I have always liked to run to one degree or another, but the only reason I can do it now and have so much fun is because of running barefoot. Living barefoot had a big impact on this, too, which everyone can do a lot more than is the cultural norm. Being barefoot makes a person feel younger on multiple levels by making movement more fun, more safe, and more natural.

I was a sprinter of sorts beginning in grade school and for a couple of years on the high school track team. While attending college, I ran a few miles each morning for fun. In the midst of raising our children, I ran off and on, a short race here and there, but not very much. Since I started running predominantly barefoot a few years ago, I have run much more. I have participated in some "official" events every year, including three half-marathons and one full marathon. I have also competed in a few sprint triathlons, finishing in good standing for my age group.

The times when I have decided to put something on my feet it has not been anything like common running shoes. In fact, I now go barefoot almost all of the time; not just when running. People who know me now tease me when I put on any foot coverings.

This book is born out of the joy I have found in running and being barefoot. I get excited to help others understand the benefits and fun of it. It does seem a little odd that it is not more normal. There is no explanation needed to understand that eyes work better if uncovered, or ears if unplugged. No serious scientific studies are done on whether or not we should all wear straightening leg braces or bind our chests so we won't breath in everyday air too deeply. However, most people are not used to being barefoot. The majority of them are intrigued and have many questions, but struggle to sift through perceived social expectations, misconceptions about foot health, and even local laws. I hope this book is useful to those who would like to free their feet.

All the usual suspects

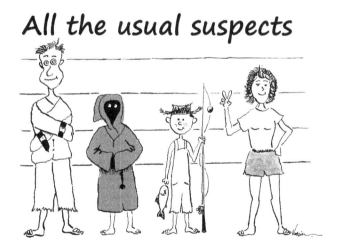

How I Decided to Run Barefoot

I wish I had discovered barefoot running sooner in my life; however, in retrospect I believe my enjoyment of running as a child was discovered prior to the development of the stiff and padded running shoe. As I remember, the earlier, pre-waffle versions of athletic shoes were much more minimalist. It was with them that I learned to love running. I don't remember buying shoes described as designed for running until I was an adult and "could afford such a luxury." I was so disappointed by my first run in them. I thought it was because I was "getting older." I don't think that anymore.

In spite of that disappointment, I kept trying to run in between pregnancies and tiny babies. Sometimes it was more fun than others, but most of the time it just felt hard. Hard to get going and hard to keep going. I liked the way my lungs and circulation felt refreshed afterwards, and that is what mostly kept me going. Sometimes, though, I wondered why I didn't just stop running and go for walks, like I was beginning to see other people "my age" do. Then, injuries began to complicate my life. Some were not directly due to running, but impacted my ability to continue to run.

One day, in a state of emotional turmoil, I wrenched my knee while gardening. Surgery helped fix the damaged meniscus. Then, at about age 45, I began to have a lot of trouble with one of my iliotibial bands. This long band of tissue, that runs on the outer aspect of the leg, was causing me pain on the outside of my knee. I tried everything, from strengthening to stretching to being careful about running around curves and on sloped shoulders of roads, but it always felt bad after about a mile.

Then, my husband began researching his own issues with plantar fasciitis. He stumbled upon someone recommending barefoot running, and he casually suggested it to me. It sounded like a fun experiment. On my next run, I was shoeless, bare sole to indoor wood track that I ran on at the time. I was immediately enthralled! It was all that I remembered of childhood running and more. I was running faster and felt lighter. I ran a joyous mile.

True, I could barely walk the next day, but a little research taught me why. I had overdone it since my legs and feet were not used to that particular kind of use. It was akin to a fit cyclist thinking a mile run would be no big deal. Running barefoot uses different muscles than running in shoes.

One thing I knew for sure: I was going to continue with this "new" way of running. It was clear that it would take more time to adjust to running barefoot than I had originally thought, but that first run had convinced me it was worth the effort. Further runs confirmed this - and now I call myself a barefoot runner.

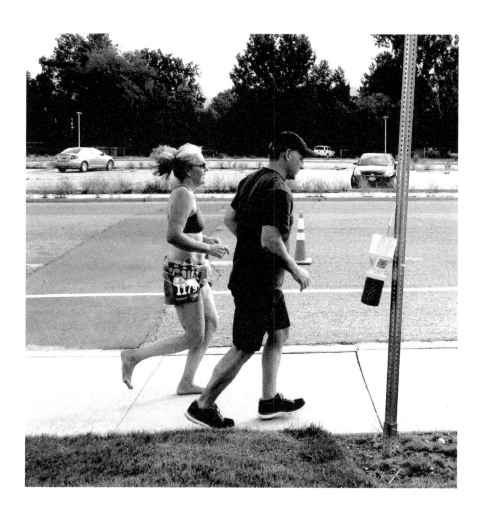

(About mile 9 of the Great Potato Half Marathon, 13.1 miles)

Chapter Two

How is the Regularly Bare Foot Different?

Health

Foot coverings may occasionally have their uses, like gloves for the hands. However, most modern shoes are more like a cast for a broken bone, or an impractical fashion statement. That is, most shoes are stiff and hold the foot immobile. Inside the average modern shoe, the network of foot bones and musculature that are designed to help a body maintain balance and gracefully absorb the shock of motion are tied up and gagged. To make things worse, for the foot thus weakened the prescription is usually more of the same confinement. Orthotics, specialized shoes, and other inserts are available to try to support the foot that has been denied the opportunity to naturally build strength. It is like putting your legs in casts, then complaining that your legs are stiff and won't walk well. Not only do the body parts get weak from lack of use, but a person is unable to perform the very movements that would make the whole body stronger.

It's not just about running. It is about overall motion and even standing comfortably. For example, since I have been living barefoot, my back takes much longer to get tired when I am on my feet for long periods, if it gets tired at all. The effect is that I don't tire as easily. This, in turn, means that I gain the benefits of added movement to my life without even really trying.

The balance benefits can hardly be overstated. If balance is not impaired, falling is not very likely. I did not set out to experiment with this, but living with a large herding dog has given me many opportunities to notice that I did NOT fall over, even when knocked into firmly or outright tripped. Besides the dog, I have been amazed at the number of times when a rug corner, misstep on the stairs, or grandchild's toy on the floor has ended with me still upright. I'm sure some of it has to do with overall strength gained from things like running and gardening. However, in such emergencies, I also can feel my toes splaying, and the lower leg muscles engaging with the partnered foot muscles. The ankle is spared unnecessary stress because of all the other joints (30 per foot) being able to function with full range of motion. There is no artificial height to hinder my balance, either, and it becomes a dance step with a happy ending. There is a good reason that bare feet are so important in the sport of gymnastics; the ability to balance is paramount to success. This insight should be applied to daily life too.

The shock absorbing function of the feet and lower legs has been hampered so long, most people don't know about it. Like any good shock absorber, when the feet are allowed to develop this natural ability, a body hardly notices it is happening. When a body is new to going barefoot, especially at a faster pace or on rougher surfaces, it might not be happening as well yet. It will take some time for the weakened structures to both get strong and more fully develop the motor skills involved, but a person new to going barefoot a lot doesn't so much have to think about it, as go a bit more slowly and give the body a chance to learn.

The feedback from the soles is more than how sharp things might feel underneath. Information about variations in texture or slope send signals to the brain about both balance and impact. When this connection has been interrupted for a while, it probably has to be relearned, like getting back on a bike after years of not riding. You can do it, but it can feel a bit awkward at first. Then, after a while, you find yourself subconsciously adjusting your positions according to the terrain. There are fewer jolts and stresses shooting up to the knees and spine because not only are the feet buffering as only they can, but other lower leg muscles can work so much better when the foot is flexible and the muscles have been developed.

As I will say repeatedly, patience and time are necessary to gain back the lost function of most people's feet. If your arm has been in a cast for 6 weeks, you don't just start lifting 50 pound bags of grain the day you get the cast off. You gradually regain the lost strength. Since most people have had their feet in shoes much longer than that, it will probably take a couple of years to let all the parts of the foot and lower leg get strong. Mine are still getting stronger in various ways after 5 years, but the strength I have gained already is fabulous. I don't regret a minute of it.

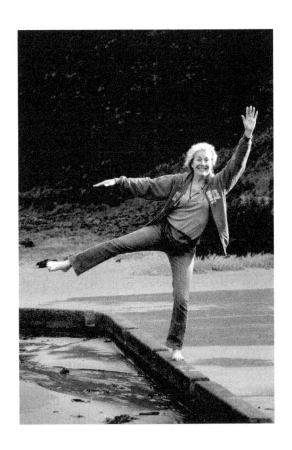

(Exploring the Oregon Coast)

What does a regularly bare foot look like?

If you take any given foot that has been confined to a shoe for the majority of its life, then let it go bare most of the time for a couple of years, it will almost certainly get wider. This depends some on the type of shoes that were previously worn, as well as if there was any barefoot time at all prior to this (such as indoors).

This widening will result from all of the muscles and bones being allowed to function as they were designed to do. Toes will splay for balance. Ligaments and tendons will have the freedom to find their natural elastic limitations as they provide shock absorption. The muscles will get stronger, which usually involves some increase in size. The foot pads on the soles will probably thicken in response to stimuli.

There will also be changes in the skin and color of the foot, both from increased circulation and exposure to air and sunlight. The parts of the skin that come into contact the most with hard surfaces will be stimulated to develop a more leathery thickness. To what degree this happens will depend on the roughness and temperature of surfaces routinely encountered.

All of this is healthy. To tell people to "wear shoes so that your feet won't get too wide" is bad advice. No one says you

need to wear stiff gloves to keep your fingers from spreading!
That would render your fingers practically useless. No one
says wear stiff leggings to keep your thighs from spreading
(we are not talking about weight gain here). To the contrary,
the leg muscles need room to flex and bend. A moderate
increase in muscle size is expected with use and is considered
an attractive sign of health.

To tell people that they need shoes so that "your feet will
stay soft" is akin to telling someone to wear a face mask to
keep the facial skin moisturized. Besides the sweat and germs,
it would be much harder to use the mouth and eyes. We
should think the same way about the feet.

Unfortunately, some barefoot advocates take these basic
facts and jump to conclusions about what a bare foot should
look like. It is not always easy to tell if a person spends a lot
of time barefoot unless you had previously examined the same
feet in question or get a chance to look more closely at the
soles. Some people's feet are naturally wider, with spaced
toes. Some people's feet are narrower. There is a lot of genetic
variation in toe length and arrangement.

The general environment makes a difference, too. You
could go barefoot all the time in the area of Taipei where I
lived for a few months and be mostly walking on smooth
surfaces with fairly constant temperatures. However, living in

rural Idaho means exposure to a wide variety of rough surfaces and weather extremes. Besides that, there are differences in humidity between the two locations that affect the skin.

The genetic aspect of foot shape could lead to erroneous conclusions, too. Photos of tribal individuals, who supposedly have gone barefoot their whole lives, are often shown as examples of what a truly bare foot should look like. There are a couple of problems with these assumptions.

First of all, it is quite possible that the shape that is assumed to be due to being barefoot is a genetic feature, like nose shape and size. Maybe the genetics of foot characteristics are tied to another feature that affected survival. It is also possible that foot shape may have made survival in a certain environment more likely. Maybe a certain foot shape was thought to be unattractive or a sign of bad omens, so the unfortunate souls were cursed or excluded. Stranger things have happened. The point is that there are numerous plausible factors that could influence the average foot shape in a given population. That is even assuming that the photos that circulate ARE even a true representation of certain people groups. To put it another way, to say that their feet look that way "because they go barefoot" is a correlation being treated as a casual factor.

Why Does Grandma Run Barefoot?

People make a similar mistake assuming that I am the shape I am because I run. The fact is that I was born with a streamlined body type. There were many years while raising kids that I didn't run. I was still the same shape. Well, off and on. It is hard to be completely streamlined while pregnant.

It is also possible that people with a certain type of feet are more likely to end up going barefoot for practical reasons. They may have a much harder time finding shoes that fit. The less culturally acceptable a foot looks, the more likely a person will seek to cover it up. These are all correlations, not causations of foot shape.

Some of my observations come from evaluating the feet of my seven children. Since they were all taught at home through high school, they spent most of their lives barefoot. True, before I had come to appreciate the advantages of going barefoot outside, I strongly suggested shoes, but they preferred going barefoot, so often did. There are some significant variations of foot type among them. Some of them have wide feet with spaced toes, but some of them have feet that taper with toes close together. Ironically, the two youngest, who have run barefoot almost as many years as I have, still have the narrowest feet of them all. These two did notice their feet widening after they had been barefoot running and going barefoot nearly all the time, but I cannot see it from looking at them.

My two children who have gone barefoot the least, mostly for reasons due to work, have the widest feet. Their feet are wide according to everyone's spectrum. Shoe salesmen have laughed when trying to help fit shoes. Fortunately, one of them can have bare feet or wear minimalist footwear almost all the time now, but the other still has strict workplace requirements to deal with.

What does all this mean to the new barefooter? First, there will be changes in your feet. Most likely, any shoes you do keep on hand will begin to feel snug. How soon or how snug will depend on how much you go barefoot and how confining those shoes originally were. Secondly, don't get concerned that your feet are not looking as "adapted" as some stereotypes floating around. Just like all hands are different, yet perform the same basic functions, most feet do what they are meant to do in spite of aesthetic variations.

Fortunately, most feet in our culture have not been deformed to the degree that they can't regain significant function and strength. What your own feet will look like as you go barefoot more is part of your own unique life experience.

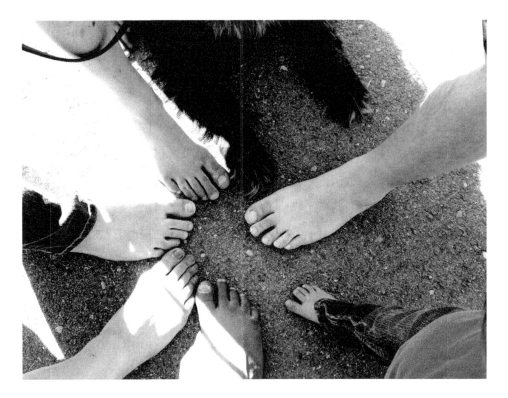

(Group photo, one foot from everyone, on International Barefoot Running Day 2016. Walkers were welcome!)

Joy

It is hardly any wonder that a person feels generally happier when movement is so much more fun! You can talk yourself out of it. You can be like a person on crutches who is sure he could never bear weight on his legs without support. You could choose to wear gloves on your hands for the rest of your life because you accidentally cut yourself with a knife once. It is your choice, but you will probably limit activities that can't be done well without bare hands, or you will greatly strain your upper body because it is not designed to handle that. The same is true for avoiding bare feet.

People often choose shoes because the style makes them happy. Possibly the advertised function promises happiness. These are good examples of "let the buyer beware." Advertising has its place - to make us aware of what is offered on the marketplace - but it should never be trusted blindly in its claims! Shoes are no exception, both in whether or not they are usually needed and how they supposedly can aide us. A "shoe" that is really helpful will allow the foot as much normal function as possible and keep movement comfortable and fun.

Too often the idea is accepted that comfort equals laziness or low-class, and because of that we don't feel free to embrace the happiness of comfort. In days gone by, women who dared to wear pants for functionality and comfort were looked down upon. I'm glad that was figured out before my time! Such a change in accepted wardrobe highlights that there is often a deeply seated, but unfounded, cultural bias against something that is inherently practical and can, in fact, be quite feminine. While there is nothing wrong with enjoying something that is substantially decorative, like earrings or hair styles, decorations that cause dysfunctional malformations to body parts (i.e. stiff, non-foot shaped shoes) should be questioned.

The rise of bizarre shoe shapes must be partly due to the fact that it was a sign of wealth to be able to afford items that are basically non-functional. Along the same lines, if there was enough money to hire out for all the physical labor you needed done (forgetting the benefits of regular exertion), impractical footwear and fashions of all sorts could be worn. Servants could even be hired to help put them on! Forget that corsets inhibit breathing and high, stiff collars greatly reduce peripheral vision while driving a vehicle. There were times past when obesity was paraded by certain royals because it displayed like nothing else that they had plenty to eat. Our society no longer accepts some of these signs of prosperity, but still considers dangerously high heels and pointy toe boxes a sign of style.

Some people wear shoes in an attempt to adjust their physical features. For instance, high heels visually lengthen the legs and alter posture to draw attention to the derriere. The overall visual addition to height can make a person look more slender. The effort of walking in high heels puts a strain on the calves that can make those muscles look stronger than they are. All of these things are part of the claim that high heels are fashionable. But at what price? Is it worth the other risks or the illusion of features?

It is hard to say how many people actually think they like our current, uncomfortable social norms and how many people succumb to the social pressure of perceptions. Sometimes we think we like things when we have been taught to think a certain way about them. For years, I thought the common modern shoe was normal and good, but didn't know it was also the unidentified source of trouble. I will now gladly abandon them for bare feet.

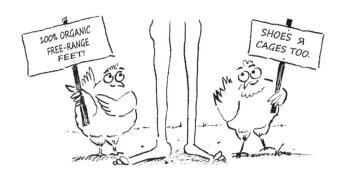

Safety

In spite of all of this information about how healthy and enjoyable being barefoot is, many people get stuck on thinking bare feet are not safe. In our culture, that is often presented as the claim of all claims, the argument that cannot be stood against. Everything has to be thought safe.

To reiterate, going barefoot provides better safety for balance and shock absorption than shoes. This means less impact to joints throughout the body, including the knees and back. The rare scrape or cut is hardly worth comparing to a bad back or twisted ankle.

There are some decisions we all make regularly, for survival and convenience. Preparing dinner with knives is not safe, not to mention heating and cooking with fire. Driving a gas-filled engine around is kind of crazy, let alone getting on an airplane. In a benefit analysis, these are what we might call calculated risks . In these instances, things with life and death risks are harnessed and utilized for the good of all.

Walking or running barefoot doesn't even come close to this. Comparatively, leaving feet bare is about as risky as breathing. Sure, there are probably things in the air that our body has to filter out. Possibly, once in a while, we run into a substance that makes us cough or sneeze. We might even, however unlikely for most of us, end up in a situation one day where the quality of the air threatens our immediate existence. Yet, we go on breathing the very natural air around us, using our sense of smell. We even use it to guide us in avoiding dangers that might hurt our whole body. We do not regularly attempt to put a barrier between us and the air. Whenever any sort of face mask is used, we like to get it off as soon as possible. It is stifling! That is how I feel about shoes!

The counter argument, why shoes are actually much more unsafe than bare feet, has already been presented some in the previous paragraphs. Wearing shoes, especially the common modern ones, is not safe. Wearing shoes with significant heels is like begging to fall over or trip, while any stiff shoes are probably already causing spine and knee trouble. It is too common that the malformations caused by shoes lead to surgical "repairs!" There are people who view their foot as the problem and have it surgically altered to fit into shoes. Then, there are all the microorganisms that grow in the dark, moist confines of shoes and smell pretty bad.

Concerns about comparative extremes in weather or terrain, will be addressed later, but be aware that what is extreme depends on experience. In the final analysis, safety concerns usually boil down to two things:

1. Misunderstanding what the supposed safety issues are, and

2. Not realizing how easy it is to deal with many perceived challenges while still safely and happily being barefoot most of the time.

Why Does Grandma Run Barefoot?

This subject will be discussed more specifically in following sections, but for now I will note that there is much inconsistency in how people apply the idea of safety. Some people act like everything can be made ultra safe. This is an illusion. Many of these same people feel no qualms about switching on electrical current in their house, but shudder at the possibility of stepping on a rock in grass. I'm not saying throw all caution to the wind, but just like I'm not going to stop dancing because I might pull a muscle one day, I am not going to stop going barefoot because something might cut my foot.

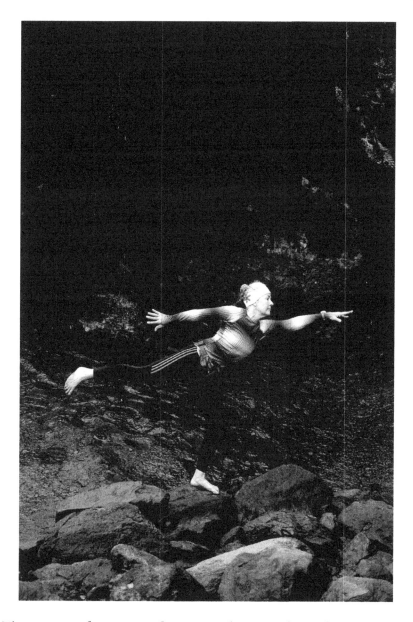

(I'm no good at yoga, but I am having fun after a run on various terrain on the Oregon Coast)

Why Does Grandma Run Barefoot?

Chapter Three

Weather, Injury, Disease, and Stigma

Most people are concerned about four things when they think about going barefoot:

1. Weather
2. Injury
3. Disease
4. Social stigma

Weather

Regularly bare feet have certain advantages in all kinds of weather. For one thing, the muscles in a bare foot are being used so much more than in a habitually shod foot. You may not be aware of how much the muscles atrophy in feet bound up in shoes, just like muscles do in any body part that is casted for an extended period. Even a stiff sandal inhibits foot flexibility in a splint-like manner. The circulation in the bare foot is much better than that of a regularly rigid foot. Good circulation helps to keep the feet and the whole body warm in winter, as well as dissipate heat in summer. (How to evaluate foot wear use in extremes will be discussed later.)

In addition to that, the skin of consistently bare feet takes on more of a skin-like character. Not being confined in moisture for hours on end, the skin is allowed to naturally toughen in a way that insulates them. There is also the simple adaptability of the body. When exposed to certain conditions regularly, the body develops its pre-installed regulatory system. If the feet are used to feeling many conditions, they will not be shocked by that exposure.

Both air and friction result in a certain toughening of the skin. When people ask to see my feet, they are usually surprised with how smooth the skin is. The soles have a smooth leather-like quality. The variety of surfaces I run on seems to buff the soles. The skin of the tops have a nice glow of pink health to them. The transition area along the edges varies with the time of year, but generally feels smooth. I hesitate to describe it as "thick," because people envision alligator skin or cow hide. It is thick the way human skin is supposed to get on bare feet to do the job it is supposed to do. One thing this conditioned skin does is keep my feet very comfortable in a variety of temperatures.

Have you ever seen someone wandering around in shorts and sandals on a snowy day and they look perfectly at ease? They are not shivering. They are not trying to make a statement. They are simply wearing what is comfortable to them in the moment. It may take a combination of adaptation and experimentation to get really good at knowing what bare feet can handle weather-wise, but it's not like people aren't doing that with the rest of their wardrobes. It's not about suffering through it and getting tough. Rather, it is about letting your feet get stronger. It is about learning what your feet are truly capable of as they are allowed to function as designed. It is about finding out that it is often both safe and comfortable to be barefoot in a variety of weather conditions.

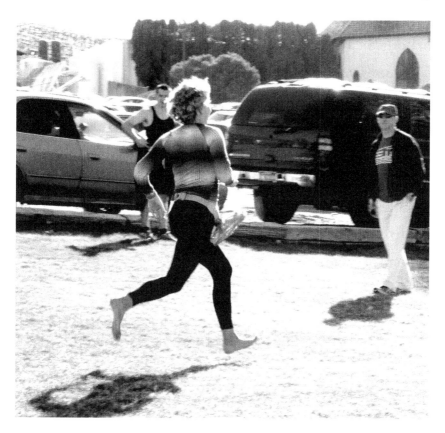

(Finishing the Shamrock Shuffle 10K on a blustery March day. Over half of the route was chip seal asphalt, some was on a dirt road through orchards)

Injury

People get hurt sometimes - even people who go barefoot. Some injuries may be unique to barefoot living, but some are unique to shoe wearing. Some people are injured because they push their barefoot training or experiences further than their bodies can currently tolerate. How detrimental that is depends on various factors.

As in other areas of life, how much trouble people think there is going to be is frequently far more than there is in reality. Also, people tend to be apprehensive about doing things differently and slow to admit the trouble right in front of them from the way it is being done now. And, people like to make up excuses to avoid things that might take them outside their comfort zone.

There are real, unexpected injuries to bare feet, but that doesn't mean going bare foot is fraught with peril, especially for someone who wants to learn how. In my barefoot history, I have accidentally run on patches of broken glass a few times without anything more than a slight nick and without spilling any blood. (Read more about that in the next section.) I have removed some skin on a stone while running when I hit it unexpectedly under a thick layer of powdery dirt. That may seem horrible to some people, but, first of all, what would they have said if I had been wearing shoes and wrenched my ankle badly? I doubt they would have suggested I stop wearing shoes. The fact is that my flesh healed much more quickly than a twisted ankle and with very few limitations on my activity.

Running in shoes often leads to blisters, knee pain, and smelly feet. People have been known to trip and fall while running in shoes. Shoes get wet and stay wet, causing even more rubbing and pain. Some tough stickers (i.e. goat head stickers that are known to puncture bike tires) and nails will go through shoes. Nails, in particular, can penetrate the shoe in a way that holds an angle to puncture the foot.

Being barefoot predisposes a person to watching for, and if that fails, feeling objects before they do significant damage. I have run in patches of sticker weeds. I won't lie. It isn't my favorite thing to do. I usually carefully maneuver to a different route, pick out any fully attached stickers, and keep running without issues. A couple of times in these last 5 years a piece of a thorn has broken off inside my foot. It was not a problem to finish my run and the piece came out one way or another easily and soon. Once, I ran with a small, white pebble lodged in a crack under a toe because I couldn't see it to remove it. It came out later in the bath, much to my surprise.

Keep in mind that I am not some tough old broad or risk taking teenager. Ask anyone in my family. I am a bit of a wimp. So, it has surprised even me that I have handled these complications with such relative ease.

Sometimes there are just accidents completely out of our control. It may mean more care needs to be taken. It could have been lack of conditioning for the level of stress on the body. Possibly it was just a quirk, but people like to be able to blame something. Anything. Too often they blame something that is illogical or convenient for their own preferences.

With all this talk of potential injury, it would be easy to forget there are a lot of nice places for anyone to easily walk barefoot - normal places a person might go every day. You would be surprised at how many pleasant pathways there are all over the world. Whether they be on man-made or naturally occurring surfaces, many are not remotely a challenge even for the new barefooter who is walking. People everywhere have a strong tendency to make smooth paths because it just makes walking easier in general.

One important way to avoid injury as a new barefooter is to gradually increase both distance and force applied to the bare feet. Walking for daily activities of life is rarely a problem, but don't expect to be able to run or hike the same distances until the feet and lower legs get stronger. Remember, they haven't been used to doing their job because they have basically been immobilized for years.

How Running Barefoot Helps Me Manage My Injuries

Experienced barefoot runners tend to keep quiet about their injuries around shod runners, because somehow every challenge is blamed on not wearing shoes. Never mind that shoes are strongly implicated in everything from blisters to knee pain, if a barefoot runner mentions any problem, people in shoes feel justified in an "I told you so" response. Particularly for newer barefoot runners, the injuries are blamed on lack of shoes, which is true only in so much as hurting an arm recently out of a cast is due to "not wearing a cast." However, sometimes injuries just happen, because that is the world we live in. It has been my experience that running barefoot often allows me to run in spite of injuries, both for enjoyment and to keep me strong as I heal.

Take my knee, for instance. I did some major damage to my left meniscus while gardening (with shoes on) several years ago. I ended up getting it surgically repaired. This really meant getting some of the cartilage trimmed out, so I was told I would have ongoing issues with my knee since the joint was now more vulnerable. Running barefoot has changed my running form to a softer impact, which is much easier on the knee.

Continued barefoot running gives every evidence of strengthening my legs in very balanced ways, ways that support knee function by engaging all the muscles surrounding it. This is probably because I am using my whole foot and not just landing hard on the one point of impact that a shoe allows. Even when I tweaked my knee uncomfortably in the garden a short while ago, I only needed a couple of days rest before I could run with absolutely no discomfort during the run and no post-run side effects.

The fact is, gardening has caused me more trouble than running, because I tend to twist and push in ways that put much more strain on my legs. Pushing digging tools into the dirt, pulling loaded wagons, or constant squats are a few examples of the motions that I engage in semi-regularly, and sometimes too much in a given time period. Barefoot gardening helps me keep these motions in the realm of balance. Barefoot running helps me work out the kinks!

Some injuries are idiopathic. I apologize, but I have loved that word ever since I first heard it in nursing school! All it means is that there is no apparent reason for a disease or injury, like the strange twinge I got in the middle of my ankle the other day during a medium long run. It was a distance I had worked up to gradually and stayed at for a few months - nothing strenuous or stressful about the pace I was going. I was running on a familiar path. I didn't trip or step on anything. It just twinged, and I couldn't finish the run that day.

I spent a couple of days not running, but stayed on my feet otherwise doing normal household and yard chores. The sensation was there off and on, but minimally as long as I didn't run. I also took my regular hot baths and put my ankle through relaxed range of motions. Over 3-4 days, I could feel whatever it was relax. The next week, I tested it with a 6 mile run and there was no problem whatsoever. Having run quite a bit in shoes in the past, I think it is unlikely I would have been able to run lightly enough in shoes to do this. The natural shock absorption of running barefoot now being well developed meant there was very little impact to my ankle.

I expect there will be other injuries in my future. I will step on sharp objects or push myself too hard during a specific training period, but barefoot running will still be fun and the best way for me to avoid worse joint injuries, as well as manage any injuries I incur.

So, I ran barefoot through crushed glass

As usual, on a particular day, I was watching for glass. I was doing this partly because I always watch where I am going, but also because a couple of days previously I had seen some glass. It had looked like freshly broken bottles. On this day, I couldn't see it, even though I knew exactly where it had been, since I had picked my way through it several times on the previous run, repeating the 4 mile stretch for a long run. So, I thought to myself, "What a great clean-up crew they have around here!"

I continued back and forth 3 more times without seeing the glass. I was running 12 miles on a section of path where I didn't have to deal with traffic except for a couple of street crossings with crosswalks. Then, voilá! On my fourth pass, there it was. Crushed glass was spread all over the path, from side to side across the whole path and for about a 3 foot long section. I would have had to step on this spot at least once with each pass through. The sky had been overcast and it seems the light had been such that the glass had been blending into the asphalt visually. Now it was quite obvious and sharp looking.

The question of glass is one of the most common concerns expressed when people see me in my bare feet. Part of my answer has always been that I watch where I am going, like - hopefully - everyone does. Another major point is that an occasional flesh wound is better than ongoing back and joint problems, not to mention fungal infestations. Still, I would rather not step on it.

In fact, that first day I mentioned going through the glass, I was trying to be careful and still got a small shard stuck into the lower side of my foot. I felt it immediately and stopped to flick it off, then I kept running the remaining 4 miles of my then 10 mile run. For the next 24 hours, I felt the shallow cut once in a while, but it only barely entered my consciousness. I was barefoot the whole time.

On this second run, I never once got any glass in my foot, whether I could see the glass or not. There was another patch that I did not relocate, but must have also run through. I have heard of other barefooters walking on broken glass without getting cut, but I had been leery. I had also heard of a couple of barefoot runners who occasionally remove small pieces of glass. Now I know from my own experience that either scenario is likely to be insignificant.

I have to think that being and running barefoot for about 3 years (as of that time) had some effect on the outcome. The toughened bottoms of my feet are not easily penetrated. I have stepped on quite a few weed stickers that only barely stick in. Once in a while, a piece of gravel breaks the skin, but the discomfort is short-lived. My feet still feel things, but it is not tender unless I am testing the limits. Rather, it is usually informative and pleasant, like a mild foot massage.

It seems I won't always see or feel glass; I may have stepped on it other times and not known it. It wouldn't be the first time that someone was afraid of something that, in reality, wasn't a big deal. Sure, glass can have sharp edges, but I think most people have picked up pieces of glass with their bare fingers without hurting themselves. Plus, there is no reason, especially on asphalt or cement, why a large piece of glass would stick up like a knife to cut deeply. Smaller pieces are apparently similar to gravel indenting instead of slicing.

Dealing with minor cuts, scrapes, and cracks

I live in a very dry, high desert climate. Even when I wore shoes about town, I had regular trouble with the skin on my feet cracking. Since going barefoot, I pay closer attention to my feet, washing them with water (too much soap washes away good oils) daily and putting olive oil on them regularly. I notice cracks and tend to them sooner too.

One way to do this is a nighttime application of petroleum jelly covered by a bandaid. Usually one or two nights of this helps the skin heal. Sometimes the crack closes, but sometimes it sort of grows new skin over the crevice.

If the crack is particularly deep or it is an actual cut, it can be helpful to cover it during the day. I have used

- duct tape
- bandaids
- medical strapping tape
- superglue

Either of the two kinds of tape can stick to the skin in uncomfortable ways, but a bandaid is often not secure enough by itself, so I sometimes use a combination of bandaid reinforced by tape. None of the tapes or bandaids consistently stay on long for running, though. The Leukotape brand medical strapping tape has done the best, but it depends on what part of the foot and how rough the surface being run on is. More and more, I find that after the first couple of steps running, I am not bothered by any cracks unless they are in a super sensitive spot or are unusually deep.

Superglue is somewhat controversial. Some people are concerned about it being absorbed through the skin or open cut. I have not found any information that convinces me that this is a real problem. I am comfortable using it occasionally over smaller cuts, or in places where tape simply will not stay put. It dries fairly quickly. My main frustration with superglue is the tubes drying closed after one use!

The fact is, that for all the miles I have run barefoot, I have had very few cuts or scrapes. Certainly not any more than people get from shoes rubbing them raw. And no more than people get from using their hands as intended. The more I let my feet do their job, the better things work out.

Disease

The way people talk about bare feet getting dirty or coming into contact with germs, you'd think people never touched anything dirty with their hands. The fact is that skin is a very good barrier for keeping out disease-causing microorganisms. That is why nearly all of us simply take care with washing our hands when necessary, as opposed to constantly wearing gloves. We are careful about what order we touch things. We are careful about touching sick people. When we have been in a public place, we usually wash our hands when we get home.

If you have ever taken care of a wound, you know that letting it air out is an important strategy for avoiding infection. There is something about a healing area being exposed to air that inhibits growth of pathogens. Keeping a part of the body moist and warm, like under a bandage or in a shoe, creates the perfect kind of places for germs to grow.

Bare feet have the advantage of constant airing out. The increased circulation, due to the foot muscles being used more completely, means that white blood cells are passing by regularly to combat any invaders. Bare feet also benefit from quite a bit of comfortable friction on most outdoor surfaces. This is not the sort of friction that creates heat or pain, assuming a person is being wise about their transition to barefoot life. It is friction that imperceptibly scrubs the soles. Lastly, feet that are allowed to be bare on a regular basis have leathery soles, not easily penetrated by unwelcome substances. My feet actually look pretty clean after a run on asphalt, but when they do get really dirty, I just wash them. I also give them a regular end-of-day washing, right before I climb into my nice, clean sheets.

Of course, I am speaking of normal, average situations. At the risk of repeating the obvious, sometimes people choose to wear gloves for protection from excessively dangerous materials. However, it is not normal to want to wear gloves all the time. I might add that people can get a false sense of safety from wearing gloves, thinking the gloves block things they don't, or not being as aware of the order they touch things to keep from spreading germs (I have witnessed this on more than one occasion). And gloves always hamper dexterity of finger function. Many people have worn shoes so much, they don't even think they need toes!

Can You Catch Cold from Running Barefoot in the Winter?

How does a person catch cold? More specifically, does being barefoot in cold conditions increase the likelihood of catching cold? The premise seems to be that colder temperatures lead to illness. However, in the case of the common cold or influenza, the only real clear factor is invasion of pathogens, specifically viruses. Even with that definite factor, not everyone gets sick or shows symptoms to the same degree, so there must be other variables.

Some stresses seem to lower a body's resistance to fighting off germs, but even those stressors are not clearly applicable to everyone. For instance, being excessively tired is thought to predispose one to getting sick, but it is also a phenomena that sometimes a parent will not get sick when their kids are suffering in ways that require significant care. I have had this happen to me when one person after another in the family came down with a prolonged delirious fever. Through no mental powers of my own, I remained healthy for several weeks and was able to care for them, even though I was quite tired from the effort.

Lack of proper nutrition, or food of questionable spoilage, are thought to lead to sickness. There again, it seems to depend. My husband seems to be able to eat anything and not get sick, whereas I have unpleasant repercussions from food that is even slightly old. Overall, though, I tend to eat a more consistently nutritious diet, but I have always gotten any germ more easily than he has.

It has been this way for all the 30 plus years of our marriage, and I have only been going barefoot for around 6 years. I might even be getting sick less often since I've been going barefoot, possibly because of all the deep breathing of miles and miles of barefoot running!

To say that exposure to cold causes illness has one major problem. Cold is a subjective sensation. It is moderated by such things as body mass, activity level, and adaptation to climate. We have all seen the person from the tropics wear a parka in mild winter weather in a region where the long-term residents are still wearing shorts and flip-flops. Then, there are the times when we go outside dressed in layers of warmth, only to strip them off for comfort as we generate heat from chopping wood or skiing. Does it stress the body to have the pores open, sweating to get rid of excess heat? Would it not rather stress the body to not let it cool off when it obviously needs to?

To be thorough, let's ponder whether or not exposure of any certain body part is more likely to stress the body. Do bare feet touching the cold ground stress the body so that germs can overpower the immune system? Would this be more of a stressor than the nose breathing in relatively cold, but not painfully frigid, air and needing to warm it? Is it worse than the hands being exposed or the head being uncovered if the body is in balance with the outdoor temperatures by either other clothing or activity?

With all the increased muscle use and better circulation of well-used bare feet, more heat is produced to keep the feet warm. As mentioned previously, the tougher skin and developed padding also insulate. Without the moisture saturating a foot, the way it does inside of most shoes, warmth is more easily retained. Plus, being barefoot tends to help a person be more active since it is comfortable and increases balance. This activity increases circulation throughout the body and stimulates fuller breathing, which cleans out the lungs and boosts the immune response. In view of all of this, it seems that going barefoot regularly could help fight colds!

Stigma

The biggest problem with stigma is what you perceive it to be. Although the occasional difficulty in a store or hospital may be embarrassing or confrontational, most of the time people don't look at your feet. If they do, they are curious, especially if you are also wearing your diamond earrings… got to keep them guessing!

If you take time to know what laws there are and aren't, you will be better able to handle issues when they arise. Laws requiring footwear are practically nonexistent; and they are almost always for employees, not customers. It is not difficult to deal with a question now and then. You should be able to go about bare footed with hardly a second thought. It is so normal to me now that I frequently forget I AM barefoot until I get a reaction. Reactions are usually anywhere from incredulous to "that really makes sense."

This is one of the areas where being socially connected to a barefoot group can come in handy. There are experienced people in these groups who can show you how to figure out laws in your area (which are usually non-existent), give advice about how to deal with naysayers, and provide examples of how they go about their normal barefoot lives. There may be a lot of new barefooters in such groups who tell upsetting stories, but keep in mind that the traumatic often gets more air time than the mundane. Also, there is sometimes confusion or disagreement about politics and discrimination (i.e. should there be laws that force private property owners to allow barefootedness).

Out of the many odd ways people choose to present themselves in public, being barefoot is one of those that people feel most free to comment on. Sort of like some people feel free to tell others they have too many children. You can be bothered if you want, or you can roll with it. Set the boundaries of your discussion, but recognize that you are going have encounters. People people-watch for all kinds of reasons. Some of them comment. It is up to you how to respond to them.

Since going barefoot is not that common, I find that people frequently want to ask honest questions. The trouble with this can sometimes be that it is a constant interruption. I currently try to judge how interested a person really is in using the information and balance that with how much time I am willing to take in the middle of shopping or running or vacation. Sometimes I answer briefly, but refer them to my blog (funfitnessafter50.com) or the Society for Barefoot Living. If the person begins to circle around to explaining all the reasons they "can't" go barefoot, it is fairly evident that there is no real interest in facts. None of us needs to be captive to someone else's curiosity.

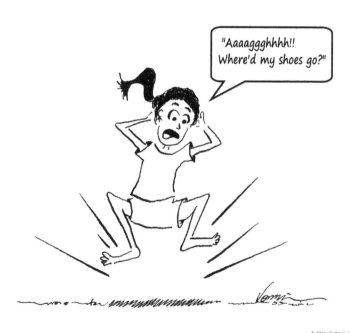

Why Does Grandma Run Barefoot?

Chapter Four

Learning to be Barefoot

What About a Scientific Study on Barefoot Running?

Learning about being barefoot does not have to be complicated. One of the biggest hurdles is overcoming years of being told shoes are necessary. Suppose someone told you that there is a scientific study showing that people should protect their eyes from light all the time. The reasoning might be along the lines that: Since we shouldn't look directly into the sun, light in general must be risky. If this became popularly accepted by most people, darkening glasses might become normal. Soon enough, there would be a variety of fashions to choose from. Manufacturers would come up with models that darkened the best, while still claiming to provide the best vision possible.

Pretty soon, people would be so unaccustomed to seeing each other's eyes that if someone didn't wear darkening glasses, it would be thought rude or too personal. After all, everyone would know that you only take off your darkening glasses in the privacy of your own home. No matter that there was a long list of injuries from people running into things or not being able to communicate well. The next glasses on the market would take care of that. People would be certain that the upcoming scientific discoveries and technological break-throughs would help with these issues.

This is not so far-fetched. People are good at coming up with alterations on human form that often do more harm than good. Corsets are even now making a comeback, even though they inhibit breathing, cause digestive issues, and lead to malfunction of abdominal organs. But, hey, they are stylish!

There have been a number of studies released about whether or not barefoot running is good. I have read many of them. As with most so-called scientific studies, there are many important questions to ask about the results. However, I think the most important questions are along the lines of:

- Do you need a scientific study to tell you that bending your knees when you walk is helpful?
- Is it good to wear noise reduction devices over your ears all the time to reduce risk of injury to your ears?
- Should your neck be held in an immobilizing brace while you move, to avoid any possible stress?

You get the idea. We know that inhibiting movement or sensory input would greatly limit functionality of these body parts. The end result would be weakening of them from disuse, and probably injury both from trying to accommodate the strange limitations and because they are now weaker.

We might want to wear earplugs once in a while. It might be good to support our necks during an amusement park ride. There might even be times to brace the knees for a unique situation. But these are all exceptions and due to unusual circumstances.

There is a reason that gymnasts go barefoot. There is NO footwear that can give them the same balance and flexibility that being barefoot can. There is NO footwear that allows the same powerful use of their legs. They need the spring of the unshod foot. They need the splay of the toes. The human body is designed to interact with the environment in ways that cannot be mimicked or enhanced by shoes, gloves, or clothes. When protection is used, it always limits the interface and experience.

Normal running and walking are basic human movements. The body is designed for them. These motions differ from activities like riding a bike or skiing, where equipment is used to allow the body to do something it cannot do on it's own power or mechanics. Running and walking are the default means of human locomotion.

As such, there should not be any need for a study to prove that using the feet fully and unhindered is best for either running or walking. There shouldn't need to be a study to show that the less interference with foot function, the better. If some sort of protection is desired at various times, it should mimic the natural foot. Just like with any other aide device, the goal should be to provide an amount of protection with the least change of function and most perception maintained as possible.

In fact, there have been studies that clearly show the damage and distortion that shoes cause, but these are generally ignored. Wearing high heels is still not controversial in most circles. On the other hand, I can not find any creditable studies concluding that people should wear shoes most of the time.

If you want to be even more savvy about evaluating studies, you can ask other revealing questions:

How large was the sample size tested?

How did they set up a control group?

What is the researcher's experience and own personal choice?

Who is paying for the study?

How significant is a test of people doing something they have never or hardly done before?

What, exactly, is being measured?

What was the environment for data collection?

What other variables were involved and how were they accounted for?

How were the questions phrased and who asked them?

How did they take their data and synthesize it into the conclusion?

If you take a group of people who have been wearing darkening glasses for their whole lives and ask them to function with bare eyeballs out in the sun, they will have a number of problems! Though at first they may find it invigorating and beautiful, they will likely get sun damage from too much exposure too soon. They may find the glare overpowering and not know how to moderate it. They might get overwhelmed by the stimuli and just say it hurts their eyes. How well they adjust will probably be affected by things like their age, the comments and reactions of people around them, and the strong human tendency to go back to old habits. If they continue to go without darkening glasses, realizing the long term benefit, they will almost certainly be labeled rebels or stupid.

In all likelihood, someone would decide to do a study on whether or not it is good to go around without darkening glasses. They will find that it is not safe to walk around without them. Then, it will become an even more firmly held "fact" that darkening glasses are needed. The consensus will be that life without them is just too hard. Some people will make laws requiring them, both to protect people from themselves and for the sake of propriety. Some businesses will have signs that say "Glasses or Go Away." But a few delighted souls will continue to live in the full light of day and get to experience life more completely, safely, and with greater health.

How to Get Used to Going Barefoot

When a person gets a cast taken off, they don't put it back on once in a while as the body part strengthens. Instead, the usual protocol is to gradually increase activity and demands on said body part. Similarly, there is no reason to keep on wearing stiff, confining shoes to help transition to being barefoot. A new barefooter can usually go ahead with walking without severe restrictions. After all, what is the first thing most people want to do when they get home from anything? They want to take their shoes off! Their feet long to be free unless they suffer from some rare abnormality or they have been severely crippled by shoes.

The easiest place to go barefoot is in the house. You may find rogue stickers that have made it indoors, places where grout needs to be redone, or shards of bone the dog has left around, but it is a more controlled environment than outdoors. I have put my feet to work in the house, much like I might use my sense of smell to alert me to cleaning issues. The solution to a puddle of water stepped in by the dishwasher is not to put on shoes, but to clean up the mess.

Learning to go outside with bare feet, whether walking or running, should just be an extension of any environmental evaluations. You will need to be cautious of extremes in temperature, especially at first when you are not as good at knowing what to expect or how your feet will react. Some surfaces will be obviously more abrasive, and exposure should be gradual, but the real key is to proceed slowly almost anywhere. Learn how your grass really feels, how many potholes there are in it, where the patches of bee attracting clover are, what debris is hiding in the blades. Don't plan on spending too much time on the asphalt in the heat of summer until you have adapted. It may seem like a lot to think about at first, but it only takes a little extra thought, like if you aren't used to a desk job and need to remember to move around so you don't get stiff.

New barefooters are often tempted to stick to only soft, comfortable surfaces. It is actually better for overall development of the foot and lower leg to regularly try rough surfaces, although for short intervals at first. The rougher surfaces engage more muscles and make you stronger in a more well-rounded way. Think of a greenhouse plant that needs to gradually adjust to being outdoors. A bit of wind now and then toughens up the plant, but too much will thrash it.

There is some danger with soft surfaces, too. Such surfaces don't teach the body to moderate impact as well. Soft surfaces can lull you into not paying attention. When you are newer to going barefoot, you don't want to be lulled. You need to pay attention and learn. Going for a run barefoot on the beach might seem poetic and be fun, but you may be hurting the next day.

It doesn't take long to get a feel for how different surfaces are affected by heat, cold, or moisture. At first, the experience of feeling so much with your feet may seem odd, but soon enough you will be so used to it that putting on shoes will be like unnecessarily putting on gloves when bare fingers are the most useful. If you really need to put something on your feet, choose minimalist footwear that allows the foot to move freely inside and mimics being barefoot as closely as possible. I will outline my thoughts on evaluating minimalist footwear in another segment.

Letting the Body Learn to Run Barefoot

Running is like writing. Everyone will do it differently, but there are some basics to think about that help with the process. That being said, these things should not be concentrated on, per se, but relaxed into. The key thing is to let the body develop a barefoot form which will be comfortable, fun, and useful.

1. Let the knees bend more. You will tend to do this naturally, more in some situations than others.

2. Let the foot come into contact with the ground nearly all at once for the most common, relaxed running pace. It will want to do that if you are not forcing it otherwise. The arch tends to be more prominent toward the inner aspect of the sole, so the outer edges of the sole will have the most contact with the ground. There is a lot of talk about which part of the foot is best to land on first. In my experience, this will change some naturally with speed (which shouldn't be attempted until the steadier barefoot form has developed quite a bit). It will also depend on terrain. Overall, the foot will want the whole sole to come into contact with the ground almost at once, possibly a split second sooner with the front half of the foot. But, again, don't think too hard about it.

3. Think about running lightly. This doesn't mean spring up and down. On the contrary, that is a waste of motion. Instead, aim for running in a way that makes you feel like you are floating somewhat. Even when running more slowly, this will give the right amount of spring to your stride.

4. Change up your pace, within it's comfortable range, once in a while. This will subconsciously stimulate your brain to experiment with the best form.

5. Relax your legs, beginning with the hips. Sometimes, in an effort to try, we unconsciously tighten up the muscles that are trying to work. Let the tightening and relaxing happen naturally with movement, but let them relax in between. This is similar to how swimmers are taught to relax the arm on the return stroke above the water.

6. Stay within a comfortable breathing range. When we are out of breath, we tend to flail and pound, basically in a survival reaction to just get done. This destroys good, relaxed running form.

7. Learn when to lean. Specifically, try a very slight lean into the forward direction from the middle of your body when on level ground. When running uphill, lean forward some, the amount depending on the angle of the hill, from the shoulders, bending a bit at the waist. When running down hill, tilt slightly back and bend the knees more, but do it in a relaxed way.

8. Remember that form deteriorates when we get tired. It also gets harder to pay attention to our environment. This will make you more prone to injury, and likely to develop bad habits. Instead, make it a habit to not push past your limits very far. Little by little, you will get stronger and your outer limits will be more impressive.

Running will come more naturally without shoes, especially if you don't try to hard. There just needs to be some time to unlearn bad habits from shoe wearing and let body parts get stronger.

How to Test and Extend Barefoot Abilities

No two people have the exact same experiences in life. For this reason, there are no set rules for how to test and expand barefoot abilities. However, there are some guidelines that are very helpful to avoid hurting yourself before your feet and legs have gotten stronger.

1. Walk or run more slowly than you usually do, at least for a while. This will accomplish two things. You will avoid injury because a more appropriate form of motion can readily

develop; and you will have more time to evaluate where you are going. It is normal for your cadence and stride to change. This is not weird. It is your body doing what it needs to do for proper balance, low impact, and maneuverability. After some adjustments, you will walk more smoothly and graciously than is possible in shoes.

2. Begin with very short periods when trying any new surface or temperature that is not close to your known range of ability. Just like a sunburn doesn't always become obvious until it is too late, damage to weak feet can sneak up on you. Such setbacks are frequently only annoying, but can result in more extensive injury.

3. Don't worry so much about your feet being dirty. While there is dirt on the ground, there is probably worse stuff growing in shoes. Not only that, but as the foot's skin toughens in all its good ways, stuff won't stick or permeate the skin like it could when the skin was shod-soft.

4. When you wash your feet, do it gently. Only use soap when really necessary, to avoid stripping oils that help keep the skin supple. This is especially important in drier climates. Also, avoid scrubbing that will remove the very toughness

that a healthy bare foot develops for its own well being. The bottoms of feet don't pick up junk like the soles and crevices of shoes do. Feet are amazingly easy to clean.

5. Avoid any foot deforming shoes. Your whole body needs the toe spread, arch movement, and flow of footfall that happens when a foot is allowed to perform its function. Wearing shoes that contort the feet damages them in ways that make it much harder for them to do their job even when bare.

6. If footwear is required for a job, a private business you want to use, or you honestly cannot deal with the barefoot conditions for the moment, find non-confining, flexible footwear. More details about how to evaluate such footwear and potential sources will be gone over later.

7. If you have had problems with foot odor in the past, the more you go barefoot, the less problem you will have, so not to worry! The fresh air inhibits growth of what causes that unpleasantness.

8. Don't compare your progress to other people's. While there are a lot of useful and encouraging stories out there, the

variability of circumstances makes it risky to just do something the way someone else is. Maybe they have had more barefoot time than you. It could be they suffer from their choices later, but you don't hear about it in time or at all. Some people just have different tolerances than other people. I know of one lady my age who won't run barefoot in the cold, but is comfortable on surfaces warmer than I can handle at this point in time. Another who definitely prefers chilly winter. They are both a couple years older than me and run faster than me!

9. When you get advice from other barefooters, remember that other newbies can be fun to swap experiences with, but their barefoot advice should be taken with a grain of salt. On the other hand, anyone who has gone barefoot most of their lives may have a limited understanding of what it takes to make such a major change.

10. Do the vast majority of your running with bare feet! However, don't switch to running the same distance with bare feet that you have been running while wearing shoes. It can be tempting to try to keep up mileage or pace with minimalist shoes, but you will be at great risk for injuring yourself if you do. The bones and muscles of feet and lower legs need to

strengthen, plus your running form needs to develop for shock absorption. Minimalist shoes mask the sensory input that would naturally limit you when you need to be limited. You don't want to end up with strained tendons or foot fractures from expecting your feet and lower legs to do what they are not capable of yet.

11. Self massage and trigger point techniques are good for any muscles that are being positively stressed within healthy limits. Make a habit of applying comfortable heat, then applying these techniques to your feet and lower legs. You will have less trouble with lingering sore muscles or stiffness.

12. Keep in mind that the range of conditions you enjoy and/or function well in will widen as you go along. However, your tolerances may vary at any given time due to various things. Some examples are:

- How physically or mentally tired you are
- Whether or not you are ill
- Unpredictable variables in speed or terrain in group activities
- How much you have recently trained to your limits and need to recover

13. It may seem harder at first to be thinking about all the stimuli your feet will experience. Like with anything new, this takes more mental energy at first. It will become more intuitive as you keep learning and one thing builds on another.

14. There is usually more than one factor to take into account when evaluating a surface. For instance, and perhaps most obviously, moisture affects perceived temperature and actual heat loss. Wind chill also does this. Less obviously, there are different colors and compositions of asphalt and cement that affect how they reflect or retain heat. How you might tolerate the roughness of a surface can be affected by temperature of either your feet or the surface. Very importantly, some types of surfaces can hide potential threats. Neither lawns nor powdery dirt should be taken for granted.

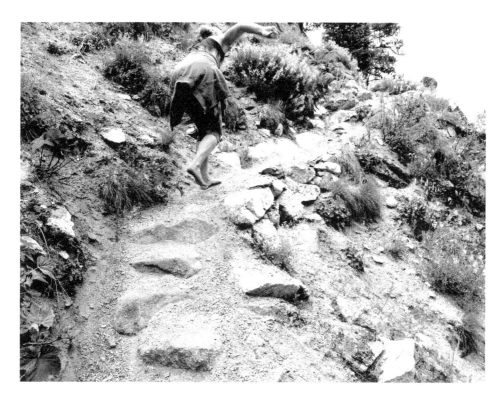

(Hiking The Crooked River Trail in Idaho. I hiked most of the time in my Moc3's, a thin Soft Star moccasin, but this hill was easier to climb barefooted.)

Why I Take a Hot Bath (and NOT an Ice Bath) for Muscle Recovery

I take a hot bath at the end of nearly every day, to both aid the recovery of my muscles after intense activity and to relax. I exercise 5-6 days a week, alternating running, swimming, and biking, as well as yard work to take care of our acre, chicken care, and energetic housework. I do not take an ice bath. Ever. I believe I have sound physiological reasons for this.

The most common reason I hear for an ice bath is "keeping down the inflammation" after an intense effort. This sounds to me like telling your body to be quiet and stop working on things because it is inconvenient for you. Inflammation is not an injury or disease. It is a symptom. More precisely, it is a mechanism that the body uses to heal itself. If the body is responding to stimuli with inflammation, in most cases it is doing the right thing to repair a section. It is increasing blood flow to an area that needs the extra blood flow.

When the body is trying to do a helpful thing, you should work with it, not against it. A hot bath (not scalding, but providing heat in a soothing way) does just that. It increases general circulation. It is pretty easy to make sure that legs get immersed. Depending on the size of your bathtub, other muscles can get nicely warmed, too. This heat helps the body move the cells and chemicals to and from muscles that need attention.

Such a bath also helps relax points of tension in the musculoskeletal frame. This by itself is good, potentially helping to avoid straining a tight spot later. It also makes a little self-massage or trigger point therapy more effective. With all this relaxing in gentle heat, the pressure applied can stimulate even greater relaxation of the body part. The pressure does not need to be vigorous or prolonged. Please research about trigger points for a more complete understanding of this.

Besides aiding in musculoskeletal relaxation, a hot bath and massage increases circulation to the extremities. Much like walking pushes blood up through the veins by action of the muscles contracting and relaxing, massage can passively increase blood return to the heart, meaning the waste products from muscle work will be cleaned up sooner. And fresher blood brings a new supply of positive factors.

Think of the body's signals in terms of pain. If something gets hurt, taking a pain killer might mask the pain, but it could lead to further damage because of not responding to warning signals. Sometimes pain killers are useful after a

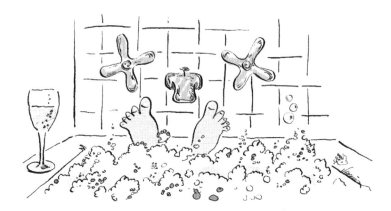

major injury, to aid rest and comfort, but we all know that continual use is bad on many levels.

There are similar issues with inflammation. Sometimes it is so bad that it may be decided to control it, but that usually involves letting the body rest and heal, too. Pain might accompany inflammation, being aggravated by the pressure of the extra fluids on the surrounding tissue. Again, this is part of the healing process, but if it is causing too much discomfort or inhibiting other healing, it might need to be moderated. However, this is not usually the case with common inflammation from exercising. A quick internet search shows that more in the medical community is coming to understand this.

Let me clarify that inflammation is NOT synonymous with infection. Inflammation frequently accompanies infection, because of its healing process, but inflammation can and does regularly occur without any infection, just due to stress on sections of the body.

And so, I work with inflammation, easing it along, encouraging circulation to the affected areas, and in doing this, I rarely have trouble with inflammation. With this approach, I don't often have prolonged muscle soreness or aches from vigorous activity, unless I have increased my exercise efforts too drastically, but even then, a hot bath does wonders. That all sounds better than an ice bath, doesn't it?

Running Barefoot in Hot Weather

Hot is to some extent a subjective term, just as we discussed that cold is. Something can feel quite hot if you are enough colder than it, to the point of pain, and still not rate as even close to dangerously hot on an objective temperature scale. Hot can seem hotter because you are tired and thirsty. You might feel the same heat with greater impact if you have low blood pressure, a certain skin condition, or are working instead of playing. You may feel hotter because of high humidity.

Realizing the subjectiveness does not mean you shouldn't pay attention to the sensation. If it feels hot to you, it may be a warning signal that the change is too sudden and fast. Still, feeling hot does not necessarily mean that you cannot adapt. Bath water that feels too hot at first can feel quite nice after proper adjustment. Sometimes you can help with adaptation to heat by doing something like providing your body with the correct liquids and electrolytes.

Some adaptations can be made on the spot, but others take time. You can quickly change into clothing that allows you to feel cooler, but many of us cannot so quickly spend time in the direct sun without burning. Adaptations for running or being barefoot in the heat also take time. Some people naturally have better heat tolerance or actually enjoy the heat, but everyone's body can get more used to it by gradual conditioning.

But before we get into that more, let's recognize that some of the troubles associated with heat and exercise are reasonably and wisely dealt with by choosing a less hot time of day. I have one barefoot runner friend who lives in Texas. He regularly gets up at 5 AM to enjoy his run. Even shod runners usually prefer to run in the cooler parts of the day, as I point out when I am asked, "But what about running when it is hot?" When I visited Costa Rica a couple of years ago, I noticed most of the runners came out after dark in the evening.

The trouble with running in the heat is that exercise itself creates heat. If the body is already working very hard to stay cool, it will not be as happy with the added stress. Within limits, however, your body can adapt to the need to do this more efficiently, just like it can adapt to increased muscle usage or the need for controlled breathing. Everyone is familiar with how muscles get stronger, but not as many are familiar with how breathing ability can improve with swimming. Swimmers aren't born with gills. What happens is that they train their lungs and circulatory system to breath more rhythmically and at longer intervals than most non-swimmers. Singers and those who play certain instruments do the same. The body is quite adaptable.

For running barefoot in hot weather, both the soles of the feet and the circulatory system need to adapt. The soles need to gradually be stimulated so that the skin there gets tough. Not all of this stimuli needs to come directly from heat. Some can come from rough surfaces, but the most specific conditioning will come from the exact stimuli. Gradual exposure to heat will be the best way to adapt to heat. It is important to note that what is felt at the moment may not adequately indicate the effect of unfamiliar levels of heat. It is always best to test new limits carefully, especially if you are new to testing those particular limits.

Speaking of the temperature of a surface, you know how in the weather report they give the measurable temperature and then the "real feel" temperature? Surfaces have their own "real feel" temperatures. The color, roughness, or materials of a surface can greatly affect how it retains heat or gives off heat. In my experience, smooth dark black is the hottest of the asphalts.

It can also make a difference what other substances are scattered about. Plant matter might absorb moisture and lend a certain coolness to the ground in the shade (where it can also hide pokey objects), but don't assume plant matter or puddles that are in the open sun are cool. If they have been there are while, or it is a particularly warm day, these substances can get quite hot, even hotter than the surface they cover. Not only that, but sometimes debris dissolves into the water and can irritate the skin. Of course, if you step into that with shoes, you have the problem of it becoming soaked into the fabric. At least with bare feet, you can just rinse and dry!

How hot a surface feels right at first is not always a good indication of whether or not your feet are ready to engage with that surface for a longer period of time, longer being relative to what you are used to. My husband had a memorable lesson in this one day when he decided to run barefoot in the middle of a warm summer day. He likes hot weather and was used to running many miles in shoes. He had occasionally run around half a mile barefoot on asphalt paths with me in the cool of the morning and he had been in the habit of running several miles barefoot on soccer fields hills, etc., so had some feel for it. On this particular run, he ran along fine for about two miles on the black pavement, not feeling more than slightly warm on the bottom of his feet. But, as soon as he stopped running, huge blisters developed, almost covering his soles. He healed fine without any long term consequences, but walking was uncomfortable for a few days. And he still prefers hot weather.

I can currently walk across asphalt parking lots when the air temperatures are in the 90's (°F), depending on the type of asphalt. I know some barefooters who regularly hike around in Arizona deserts. It all depends on what a person is used to. The first few days of hot weather seem hotter to most people. Then, the senses adjust to a new normal. Less and thinner clothing is worn. It should not be surprising that some people also choose to be continually barefoot during the warmth of summer.

Can You Keep Running Barefoot in Cold Winter Weather?

Most people begin barefoot running during the warmer months of the year. As winter creeps in , they wonder if it is safe to run barefoot in cold weather. The concern about illness was covered in an earlier section, but here the emphasis will be how to adapt to and prepare for being barefoot in the cold, both mentally and physically.

First of all, as mentioned, if the feet have been conditioned to be barefoot overall, they will have much better circulation than most regularly shod feet. This means that cold will naturally become more comfortable the more years a person goes barefoot. How tough the soles stay over winter will depend on total barefoot time and the length of time that winter conditions limit barefoot activity on normal outdoor surfaces. That being said, many experienced barefoot runners adapt to running barefoot in notably winter conditions. Here are some things to think about.

1. Everyone says "keep core heated," which means keep the main trunk of the body and any non-exercising parts sufficiently warm. For me, this begins in the house, before the run. It means silly things like remembering not to eat ice cream right before a cold run, but it also means:

- Trying to engage in some chores or activities around the house before the run to get my center heated.

- Making sure to dress warmly enough in the house for the period of time before the run. It never works out well to start the run chilled.

- Avoiding getting so warm that my skin and circulation start making changes to let off heat trying to get cool. This would mean setting myself up for quick cooling once I step outdoors.

- Wearing clothing next to my skin that doesn't collect moisture. Wool works best for me.

- Wearing clothing in layers that can be removed to avoid sweating, then turning into a popsicle.

- Wearing clothing that repels moisture from the outside, without retaining it on the inside. Again, a light weight wool jacket designed for running works best for me, but there are some very good synthetics, too.

2. Minimalist footwear can be a tool to help enjoy winter running, but the first couple of winters it will be important not to stress a body that has not fully strengthened to barefoot form. Your favorite choices in minimal winter footwear will probably change as you adapt to cold and your running form improves. Be aware of these things:

- Everyone has different cold tolerances. If you are feeling anxious about certain conditions, use it as a reminder to be careful about both time and distance attempted.

- Being barefoot as much as possible is a good goal and quite fun, but not at the price of losing toes or significant amounts of skin to cold injury.

- The winter weather is more intense and risky and longer in some localities. Don't be discouraged by comparing your winter running to people with less severe conditions.

- The dead of winter might be a good time to take a short break from running, as suggested by many trainers. Such a rest time can be regenerative.

- A little discomfort from the cold is acceptable, especially for a short time and if you are being active and your feet begin to warm up. But it is okay to err on the side of caution. Soon enough you will have more experience and be able to fine tune your choices.

- Cold plus wet can make a difference of 15°F (8.3°C) worth of tolerance for me.

- I find that my tolerance to dry cold had been more adaptable than my tolerance to wet cold.

3. The more you are barefoot, both running and in life in general, the less trouble you will have with your feet feeling cold.

- The first winter is not a good indication of how all your future barefoot winter running will go.

- In future years, you may actually find that your feet get hot in the middle of winter if you cover them too much.

- Cold can affect perception of surfaces. For me, rough feels much worse if my feet are cold.

- Being tired leads to both slowing down and cooling down. Be prepared for that at the end of longer winter runs.

- Wind speed and temperature will also impact how penetrating the cold is.

4. Have flexible goals about testing and increasing your cold weather tolerances.

- While it can be helpful to have some guidelines and goals, don't let those push you in to doing things that involve a high degree of risk. You can always go back and try a lower temperature or snow at another time, after additional conditioning and experience.

- Realize that there is no need to begin your cold weather barefoot journey in the worst weather extremes. Take advantage of any gradual changes in the weather to test and adapt. But also, be sure to take advantage of the odd balmy winter day!

- Learn from other people's mistakes, but don't feel pressured by other people's progress or stories of triumph. They don't have your body or feet. They may also have variables in climate and terrain that are not obvious.

- Unless you are extremely experienced and sure of yourself in winter conditions, carry back-up footwear with you. It may even be a good idea to have it on hand in familiar conditions, because there is always the chance of unexpected prolonged standing or the run taking longer than you thought.

- Don't be overly concerned about losing sole conditioning during the winter. There is a good chance you won't lose as much as you think, but it will depend on how long and wet your winter is. Some people use buckets of gravel indoors to keep their feet tough, but most barefooters I have had contact with don't, and it only takes them a very short time to get back to full-strength barefooting in the spring.

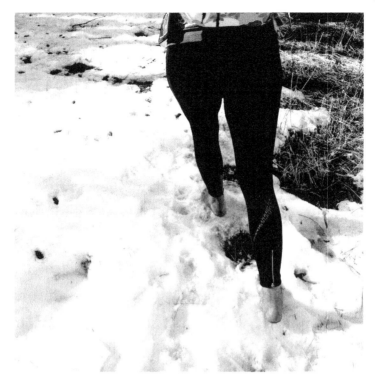

Building an Endurance Base and Core Strength

1. Build an Endurance Base

Making the change to running barefoot provides a good opportunity to re-evaluate other running philosophies. After running barefoot for a couple of years, and benefiting from the experience of others on the Barefoot Runners Society, I decided to change my approach so that I now spend most of my time running at comfortable speeds.

There are different names used for this approach, but I think the most generic is the "maximum aerobic function" approach. In a nutshell, it means letting your aerobic system gradually get stronger so that you naturally begin to run faster with less stress. Some people use a heart monitor, but I was not willing to do that. I checked my heart rate manually a couple of times, to see if I was doing a good job of keeping within a certain range, and I was.

That was nearly two years ago and I have learned to enjoy running even more by adding this to my approach. I have gradually gotten faster without the stress injuries. Combining this approach with barefoot running has been a beautiful synthesis that makes running more fun and is making me stronger with much less strain.

Recommended further reading on the concept:

80/20 Running: Run Stronger and Race Faster by Training Slower by Matt Fitzgerald

The New Rules of Marathon and Half-Marathon Nutrition by Matt Fitzgerald

Running with the Kenyans by Adharanand Finn

Why Does Grandma Run Barefoot?

<u>What Makes Olga Run?: The Mystery of the 90-Something Track Star and What She Can Teach Us About Living Longer, Happier Lives</u> by Bruce Grierson

<u>The Maffetone Method</u> by Philip Maffetone

<u>Run Less, Run Faster</u> by Bill Pierce, Scott Murr, and Ray Moss

2. Know When to Rest

Learn the difference between 1) fighting inertia or 2) your body really telling you it needs some recuperation time. These are two different problems that are solved in opposite ways. Sometimes it can be hard to just start moving on a given day, but you will feel better if you do. However, no one can workout full speed all the time. The body always needs time to adapt and recover. This not only involves adequate sleep and nutrition, but low-key days as well. Sometimes it means low-key weeks. If you feel like you are frazzled and drained, take a day or week off from intense effort and see what happens. Appropriate rest is not a sign of weakness. It is a sign of wisdom.

3. Find other types of exercise.

Running is repetitious. It tends to use the same muscles over and over. Engaging in various types of exercise is usually stimulating mentally, but it is also a good way to build a more balanced strength and avoid injury. Corollary muscles will get stronger and tired muscles will get a rest. And don't forget that just singing with gusto is good for the lungs and circulatory system. Singing can be a good way to warm up before an activity.

4. Use positive vocabulary

The words you use can have a significant effect on attitude. Instead of describing your run as "slow," speak of it as "comfortably stimulating." Never forget that "slow" is a purely subjective term, too often compared to the most outstanding effort of a professional athlete at a prime moment of time. No one maintains those moments for every run or even for a whole given year. All athletes peak and ebb, and the science of how and when that is is still being studied.

Barefoot Speed Training

Many of us want to go fast or at least feel like we are going fast. After some endurance base building and giving yourself time to adapt to bare foot running, this may be a reasonable goal. More than likely, you are really mostly racing against yourself and your limits, hopefully for the fun of it. There is nothing to be gained by injuring yourself when trying to train for speed. Here are some guidelines for barefoot speed work.

1. Don't do speed work if you are new to barefoot running. I have been running almost exclusively barefoot for a few years now. The difference in my soles and musculoskeletal structure of my feet and lower legs is important. Plus, my form is more light and relaxed than shoes would allow. The exact period of time that a given person should wait before adding speed work will obviously vary, but try it with caution especially the first few times.

2. Do a significant part of your speed work with bare feet. Minimalist footwear limits feedback that tells you that the body is hitting hard. You might be discouraged at first that your barefoot speed intervals are not as fast as those with footwear, but that will change with time and practice. Meanwhile, you will be at less risk of pounding or pulling something.

3. Do your speed training on surfaces you are used to running on and are familiar with. Your feet will be conditioned to those surfaces and your body will know more intuitively how to respond. Also, there will be less risk of hurting yourself on unfamiliar terrain, because the added speed means there is less time to observe and respond.

4. Make sure to warm up first. I usually warm up 1-2 miles before any kind of speed or hill work.

5. Cool down afterward. This helps the muscles recover by keeping the blood flowing in the muscles.

6. Keep your speed workouts fun. Sure, there will be increased and even difficult effort, but don't push yourself so hard that you will never want to do it again. Again, trying

past a certain limit will increase risk of injury anyway, which is no fun. Running with someone can be diverting in a speed workout, but don't let it tempt you to unreasonable effort. Mostly, let yourself feel like a kid, enjoying the rush of air and sense of "going faster."

7. Do not push for maximum speed often or at all. Not only will it be unmaintainable, but it won't help you that much. There may be a point at which you kick in the last few yards at what feels like top speed, but for most of us, that won't be maximum speed after even a mile or two race, let alone something longer. Not if you don't want to pull a muscle.

8. Don't try to do speed workouts with your dog. Dogs don't race by the same rules and they can turn on a dime. In an attempt to show their excitement, they may trip you or body slam you into the ground. This is not fun at anytime, but even less so while doing speed work.

9. Don't do much in the way of speed work on your longest runs. It is okay to vary pace. That is natural, and hopefully you are learning to do negative splits, with your first miles being more relaxed and getting faster toward the

end of the run. However, intense speed work during a long run is pushing too many limits in one run.

Abilities of Companions

On the whole, if you are a new barefoot runner, you either need to run with a patient, experienced barefoot runner, or you need to run by yourself. Shod runners will too often end up discouraging you or putting you in situations that lead to poor decisions. Possibly you can find a place like I have where everyone can run at their own pace, but still say hello once in a while. It is very important that you run at you own pace and comfort.

You will probably find that running barefoot is so fun, and, if you are being gradual, just the right sort of stimulation, so that running by yourself will be quite rewarding. However, even if your actual run is by yourself, there is the constant temptation to share times and compare feats. Just say no, at least for a couple of years. Let yourself enjoy your barefoot journey without all that comparing and competition. If you must compare, simply compare enjoyment and how long you stay injury free. The rest will come.

Chapter Five

When and How to Think About Minimalist Footwear

Conditions and Choices

So what is minimalist footwear, when should you wear it, and where can you get it? Broadly speaking, a minimalist shoe should let the foot function as close to how it would if it were bare. However, most people aren't used to thinking about what that means, so here are some things to consider:

1. Toe spread - If you've been wearing shoes all your life, you may have wondered why you even have toes. Toes play a major role in being able to balance. They need to be able splay apart to do this. To inhibit this splaying strains other joints further up the body when they have to compensate or because they can't. When the toes are basically bound up, the back and other upper body muscles must tighten and strain in ways that unnaturally stress them. This often leads to anything from a twisted ankle to a strained back to actually falling and

breaking a bone. This is why any footwear should have what is called a wide toe box, that just lets the toes do their job.

2. Arch function - The arch muscles need to be used, not supported. Being used will strengthen them and cure many a foot ailment. The visual of someone's arch does not indicate its health any more than shape of their jaw tells you how well someone can chew.

3. Flexibility - The best minimalist footwear will easily bend as you step, letting the foot muscles move and contract naturally with each step. While thinness of sole is not directly related to flexibility, it is a good place to begin the evaluation. However, some materials will be more flexible when thicker than others can be even if cut much thinner.

4. Ground feel - It frequently only takes a little bit of protection from rough surfaces to give the moderation desired. Try to lean toward as little interference with ground feel as possible and you will have better form in movement and more stability.

5. Sole height - It doesn't take much height added to ground level for a sole to impede balance. Center of gravity

gets moved just enough and then other joints higher up get unnecessarily stressed trying to maintain balance. A good minimal choice will add only a few millimeters to your height.

6. Grace - Going barefoot has made me observant about how shoes make people walk. Too many people think they are clumsy and clunky, when it is really the shoes they are wearing making them walk and feel that way. The best minimalist footwear will allow you to walk with the same gliding grace that going barefoot enhances.

Exactly what type of minimalist footwear you like or need will depend on the environment and your own abilities. The first year or two, you may wear something heavier during the coldest winter months. In future years, you may end up only requiring a sandal and be quite comfortable. This will also depend on how long you are out in the elements.

If you are bush-whacking through waist high sagebrush, like I end up doing on some of my adventures with my husband, you may want fully enclosed moccasins even in the heat of a summer morning. If you are going to be in unknown conditions, it might be a good idea to have back-up footwear, unless you have been going barefoot regularly in extreme

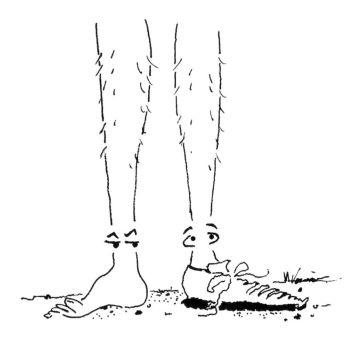

conditions and can easily keep pace with anyone you might be with.

As I stated earlier, you don't want to wear footwear unless you need to, but also don't be pressured by what other barefoot advocates do. You have to be honest with yourself about how you are progressing and how you might benefit from testing your limits, but also be honest about your limitations in situations that are beyond your current ability and experience.

Minimalist Footwear Companies

The three minimalist footwear companies that I use the most are:

Soft Star Shoes http://www.softstarshoes.com
Luna sandals   https://lunasandals.com
Sockwa   http://www.sockwa.com

Soft Star Shoes makes the most variety of minimalist footwear that I've seen. You can find footwear from them that will work for a nice restaurant that absolutely won't let you in without something on your feet (although, ironically, I find that the more upscale the establishment, the less likely my bare feet will be an issue.). And you can find footwear for running through rough terrain. I have some basic, Vibram-soled moccasins that I wear for cold weather gardening or adventuring. I have some much thinner moccasins (Moc 3's) for warmer excursions in the wild or dry, cold weather running. In the deepest, dark of winter, I am grateful to have their sheepskin lined Phoenix boots, but I wear them less every year, due to my own adaptations. One of my daughters wears the Ballerine to her office sometimes, particularly when clients are involved. She can go barefoot other times.

Luna is known for their sandals. Everyone in my family has a pair of their sandals, even if they don't go totally barefoot that much. They all like them. I have run in mine, biked in them, and danced in them. They are a good basic back-up for most casual social occasions, when I find a business owner is stubborn about bare feet. I keep a pair in my car most of the time.

Sockwas are not really marketed as minimalist footwear, being sold more as an active beach shoe. I find this amusing, as beaches are some of the nicest places to go barefoot. However, I have found the G-4 model of Sockwa to be nearly perfect for running in somewhat damp, cold winter weather for the distances I typically run (5-10 miles during the winter). I also use them for the gym, especially for weight lifting, since where I go they still require closed footwear. The Sockwas are very thin and flexible. The fabric is elastic, but not confining or squishing. Because I am usually using them in cold, wet conditions, I typically wear Injini wool toe socks with them. I do find the toe socks make a difference in how my toes work on my runs or weight lifting.

These are just my preferences for the environmental conditions I deal with, and as I try to keep up with my husband. Other people like their Altras and Vibram Five Finger (VFF) models. I tried one type of VFF's, but found they inhibited toe movement more than the other minimalist footwear I use. I think this is because the toe sections had thickish bottoms on them. I do have some totally leather VFF's that I have used for dancing, when shoes were required, and I wore them out. I have been looking at some of the VFF yoga models for possible dancing options. Other people really like Xero sandals or Unshoe sandals. You can find a lot of good discussions about minimalist footwear over at the Barefoot Runners Society, <u>but the key point is always that you must be barefoot as much as possible and increase your running gradually to develop the right form to avoid the worst kind of "too much too soon" injuries</u>.

Chapter Six

Getting Out and About Barefoot

Laws and Private Property

Laws about attire, including footwear, are generally about employees. As usual, the government thinks it needs to protect us from ourselves, so in some industries, employees do have codes to abide by or employers will be penalized. Customers are an entirely different matter. With very few exceptions, there are no laws about people just going barefoot, for anything from driving to eating out. Unfortunately, some businesses have also decided that bare feet are one thing they have to protect customers against. Ask them about high heels or flip-flops and they will either get mad or stutter and just say it is their policy. They probably sell things like cigarettes or knives, but you couldn't possibly make your own decision about bare feet. Such are the biases of our cultures.

Some businesses outright lie about laws requiring customers to wear shoes. Others are just ignorant. Still, there are a fair number who either will not harass a barefoot customer or who will listen politely to reason. Even if the business has a proven acceptance of bare feet, you can get the occasional misinformed employee who will be hard to get along with. Most of the time, a brief "I'm fine, thanks." will suffice. I have had recurring trouble with an employee in a store where being bare foot was clearly allowed. After attempting on a few times to answer nicely, I chose to ignore him. My next time in, he tried a linebacker move, but I went around. He must have complained to someone and been told his mistake, because ever since, he has quietly let me by. Sometimes you will get more trouble from the other customers than anyone, but that is how people are about anything. Some people like to find things to make fun of or complain about.

Outside is generally not an issue with anyone, though I have heard of the police being called to question a barefoot runner. Sometimes people just aren't sure if a barefoot runner is okay, though the occasional person seems to think it is an indication of criminal intent. It does depend on whether not the area is private or government run. Don't be confused about "open to the public for business." It is not the same as public property.

There is some confusion and disagreement about private property versus government-run (so-called "public") property. Government officials seem to be just as likely as private businesses owners to arbitrarily prohibit bare feet. In government cases, there is at least the appearance of being able to appeal as one of the "public" they ostensibly serve, but often people in such positions of power like to be able to tell others what to do.

On private property, the owners should be allowed to have their own opinions and standards, but you are also usually free to do business somewhere else. Unfortunately, with there being relatively few life-style barefooters around, some business owner might not care. There are many reasonable people, though, who respond well to a polite and informative explanation.

Guiding the Conversations and Concerns

Responding to questions or confrontations about having bare feet takes some practice. Too many times in the past I have felt trapped inside the box of their assumptions, trying to fight my way out. A few people will declare it to be illegal or disgusting. Now, I often simply assume the person doesn't know what he is talking about, and say in a kindly way, "Thanks, I'll be fine." More often than not, that is the end of it. If they want to go on about it being dangerous or dirty, I have to work harder at evaluating them and the situation. Sometimes just another positive statement, such as, "No, it's not. If you want to know more about it, you can go to (fill in the blank, see resources at end of book) for information." That puts the burden of research on them.

When I'm out running, one of the most frequent questions is some version of "doesn't that hurt?" I usually try to answer with a simple, "No, it's fun." and keep going. Recently, one gentleman asked me a friendly, "Where do you get your feet re-soled?" I was able to quickly respond, "Ha! They just keep getting better." He laughed, so I think he got the point.

If there is any sign that a person might give barefoot running a try, I make sure to mention starting with very short distances. Especially if said person has just seen me run 8 miles while they were fishing. It is too easy for people to forget about patient training. If I am done with my run, and have time, I am more than glad to talk about it for a while. I have discovered that sometimes I am just a curiosity and there is no serious interest. If this is the case, I don't feel guilty about getting on to more important things in my life. Of course, I can refer anyone with a real desire to learn to my blog: funfitnessafter50.com.

Dancing Barefoot in Public

My husband takes me out dancing regularly and I dance barefoot in public. We prefer good old rock-n-roll dance music, so totally free form and nothing fancy. We are usually the first ones out on the dance floor.

Not only does my aerobic conditioning from running, biking, and swimming mean I have lots of energy to dance, but dancing in bare feet means I can try all kinds of fun moves without falling down. Other customers, whom I have never met before, frequently come up to comment on how much fun it looks like I am having and they wish they could dance like that. I point out the two most important factors: running to stay fit and being barefoot.

It is always rewarding to see a few other people take off their shoes and dance. As with many things, someone has to be the first one to brave the potential social reactions. I have never had another customer in a bar or dance club complain about my bare feet. I have had many people tell me at the end of an evening how much I inspired them.

As far as these business establishments go, there are only three places out of around 30 that I have tried around the globe where the owners have said I cannot dance barefoot. Their concern for foot injury is ironic, considering they are serving alcoholic beverages whereby quite a few people are obviously affected. Some of these people even occasionally fall down on the dance floor. They probably wouldn't fall down as easily if they were barefoot! Plus, the potential injury from falling down or any other side effect of drinking alcohol is much higher than from just being barefoot. Once again, we see rules of safety and concerns for liability being weirdly skewed for reasons that have nothing to do with real probability.

This doesn't even take into account the people dancing in high heels, which is very unbalanced and dangerous, or flip-flops, which is insane. On the whole, the more upscale a business, the less problem they seem to have with my bare feet. In this I include stores and restaurants, as well. I guess they feel they have their image well in hand, plus allowing personal freedom can only help their public image. I agree with them on that.

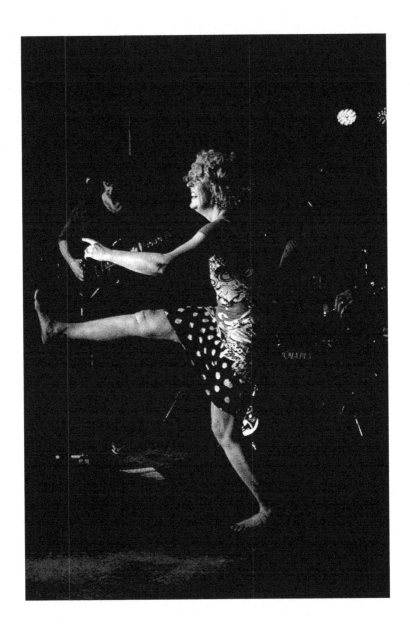

Why Does Grandma Run Barefoot?

Chapter Seven

Running Races Barefoot

Free to Choose Barefoot Running

People are purposefully and successfully running races with bare feet all over the world. This includes both men and women, of various ages and at a wide range of speeds. They do it in different climates, on many kinds of surfaces, and in assorted weather conditions. Some of them are experienced by many years, and others are relatively new to barefoot running.

There are very few races that currently require footwear, but you should read through rules of the event to avoid unexpected issues at race time. I know people who have run the New York Marathon barefoot, but apparently events put on by Disneyland require shoes. I, myself, have never been approached by a race director about running barefoot. When I have felt the need to check on a race farther from home, I have been made to feel very welcome.

However, don't forget that it is not necessary to run races to be a barefoot runner. You don't have to prove anything to anyone else, and you can enjoy running without competition. The race events can be fun and/or useful goals. They can also be enjoyable social events. It is all up to you.

Feet Before the Race

There is frequently a lot of standing around at the beginning of a race. If it is in chilly conditions, a barefoot runner may have to judge the need for pre-race foot warming. There are various ways to do this including a) more pre-race movement, b) picking a waiting area or position that helps retain heat, or c) using some minimalist footwear to retain heat. However, the well conditioned bare feet will have less trouble with this, as mentioned in previous sections.

Wear and Tear of Increased Effort

There is almost always a higher level of effort during an event, making you more susceptible to pushing yourself in ways that lead to injury. This happens to barefoot and shod runners alike. For barefoot runners, the wear and tear can be on the soles if form deteriorates or surfaces are encountered that one is not prepared for. The tendency to run somewhat faster can also lead to unexpected blisters or scrapes, especially if it is for longer distances than those speeds are normally maintained. This is because at different speeds, the bottom of the foot is engaged differently, both in surface area used and pressure exerted. All of this really just means that one should both train for the race, and then stick to racing according to the training as much as possible.

The more runners there are on a given course, the harder it can be to see where you are placing your feet or to adjust footfall quickly. The more experienced one is at running barefoot, the less of an issue this is, because running tends to be more intuitive and all surfaces are more adjusted to. The one thing that I have not heard of any barefoot runner having trouble with is other runners stepping on their toes, much like I have not heard of shod runners stepping on each other. Sure, there can be some jostling, but, actually, the tighter the crowd, the smaller strides everyone seems to take, so feet are even more directly underneath.

The terrain and roughness of race courses can be unpredictable. Unless you have thoroughly tested it or are a seasoned barefoot runner, it may be best to carry some sort of back-up sandal or moccasin. This can save you from difficult and disappointing situations. Sometimes, just knowing you have the back-up is all the mental support you need. Other times you may just slip it on for a few yards of particularly sharp terrain.

During the Race With People

Fellow racers and spectators can have strange reactions to seeing someone run by in bare feet. Most people will be positive and curious, though some will come right out and call you stupid (while you pass them). A fair number of people just want to comment for the entertainment of all who may hear, not realizing you have heard those same comments more times than you can count. You are under no moral obligation to explain your decision to everyone, anymore than everyone else needs to explain their shoes and other race gear. If, however, you find it diverting and fun, go ahead and talk to them.

Chapter Eight

I Said I Would Never Run a Marathon

I had said I would never run a marathon, and I meant it. Although I liked to run, a marathon sounded too hard. After a few years of barefoot running, I shocked myself by realizing I had changed my mind. So, I started to prepare.

It seemed wise to work up to that distance. By the time I had made the decision, I had gradually increased race distances from always running the 5K distance to entering a couple of 10K events and finally a 13.1 miler, or half-marathon. I had run one of the half-marathons in minimal moccasins, except for the last two miles. Then, I had run the same event a year later completely barefoot. Being barefoot was more fun. By then, I was ready to take on a marathon.

Really, for me the hardest thing about running the marathon was the time it took to train, not actually the effort of the training itself. There were training days that didn't go as well as others. I bonked pretty badly around mile 10 of one of my longer 22 mile runs after having worked up carefully to that distance, but I came back the next week like it had never happened. There were also training days that were fabulous, where I felt I was floating and Olympic. Most training left me feeling invigorated and optimistic.

I ran about 90% of the marathon barefoot, choosing to put on my Luna sandals for two short segments, around miles 15 and then 17, to run over sharp, chip seal asphalt. But in the last few miles, being barefoot allowed for a spring to my step, small though it was, that footwear would not have allowed. Here is the whole story, as I wrote it right after the race:

The 90% Barefoot Marathon

Here are two important lists related to this first ever marathon that I ran, and ran 90% barefoot, on Sunday, October 12, 2014. These lists are a summary of the challenges and advantages I had going into the City of Trees Marathon in Boise, Idaho.

Challenges:

- It was my first official marathon.

- I had not been able to run the course ahead of time to determine barefoot level.
- I knew I was quite likely to be facing about 5 hours of running.
- I had strained my right lower leg 6 weeks prior to the race, then my left quad about 3 weeks before.
- My mom had been diagnosed with aggressive brain cancer about 2 months before the race and I was devoted to spending a lot of time caring for her and helping my dad.
- My mom, whom I was very close to, died exactly 1 week before the race.

Advantages:

- My husband is a very supportive and wise coach.
- The rest of my family was also very encouraging and helpful about scheduling what training I could while my mom was sick.
- I have 4 years of barefoot running experience.

- I have been implementing a maximum aerobic function (MAF) approach to my training for a year, and this has made my running efforts much more comfortable.
- I have a spin bike in my basement and a swimming pool with a current generator in my backyard for alternative training.
- I have previously run some races barefoot, including the Shamrock Shuffle 10K and the Great Potato 2014 Half Marathon this spring.
- I have run 2 complete half marathons, one half in minimalist running moccasins (my Moc3's), and the half marathon I mentioned above.
- I had run several long training runs completely barefoot, including one 26.2 miler before my leg difficulties.
- I have run in extreme weather conditions of both hot and cold.
- Hills were part of my training runs now and then throughout my training, although never something I worked "hard" on.

- I had lots of good advice and support from my Barefoot Runners Society (BRS) friends when I asked for specifics related to my situation.
- The weather was perfect on race day.

I was so very grateful for the cool, sunny, dry weather on race day. It meant that most of my pre-race warm clothing could be left behind. The pre-dawn temperatures were around 48°F, and were supposed to make it to 50°F early in the run. I knew I could comfortably run barefoot, with shorts and a long sleeve t-shirt in that weather. My husband/coach, Wild Greg, advised, however, that I sit down for the half hour I had before the race, which turned out to be a good idea, as I could alternate between putting my bare feet up on my daughter's or his lap. It was pointed out to me that they were not offering to snuggle my feet under their shirts, next to their bare bellies, but I appreciated what they were willing to do.

Still, stepping outside the door to run in those temperatures is a little different than sitting around barefoot in those temperatures. I knew I wasn't risking any extremes, but I wanted to see how my feet would hold up if they got a little chilled before the race, so I didn't bring any warming minimal footwear. I had my Luna sandals in a grocery bag, tied to my water-bottle belt, for back up while running. They would have given me some insulation from the cold ground, too, but you have to admit that warm laps were better.

I had had plans to sew a pouch for my Lunas, but the last 2 months being what they were, I never got to it. It is still on my agenda. I have run with my sandals tied to me in a grocery bag many times without any trouble. They have stayed put and quickly become unnoticeable as I run, but this time they worked themselves loose, so that I ended up carrying them in my hands most of the way.

Although my feet were slightly numb from the cold for the first 3 miles, it was not enough to inspire donning of footwear. I was enjoying being barefooted and I could feel the ground. It is true that before the race, I had vacillated greatly about whether or not to just wear the Lunas. I was mentally stressed out about what kinds of surfaces I would be facing at a distance that was going to be a true test for me. Somehow, just knowing the decision was totally up to me, that there was no shame in doing whatever worked for me, helped me relax. Then, I was able to recognize that I would really be the most comfortable the more I was able to run barefoot. So, I started barefoot, but ready to do what I needed to along the way.

The first half of the race I barely glanced at my Garmin, just to notice that I had almost gone 3 miles, 5 miles, 8 miles. I didn't look at my pace. I noticed my feet were warming up nicely, but that the blinding rising sun was making it harder to see what was on the ground in front of me. I had been practicing landing more on my whole forefoot, so as to spread any landing force on gravel across my whole foot. This was suggested in another BRS forum thread I had read and when I tried it on training runs, it helped. I was not feeling any discomfort on the bottoms of my feet as I ran through some of the roadside gravel that seems to spread thinly across the road.

About the 5 mile mark was the first time my husband/coach showed up alongside me for a couple hundred yards. He was driving his car from spot to spot, taking photos and jogging alongside me encouragingly, even chatting with the other runners. He pointed out to me that his calculator brain *(my description, not his)* had determined I was running about a 10:15 minute mile pace. This surprised and concerned me. That was a good 1 to 1.5 minute faster per mile than I had been doing on my training runs since my leg problems. Since I didn't feel at all like I was exerting myself, I decided to just enjoy myself and run "how I felt." I was pretty sure I would slow down later, so why not take advantage of my floating fleetness for the time being. I wasn't breathing hard, like many of the runners around me, and my legs felt great.

During the first few miles, I met a massage therapist running her second marathon. She works in a local hospital and gives massages to mom's right after child birth. This has included a lot of refugees, so she has seen a lot of feet that have gone bare for many years. She commented to me how leathery they all are, and I could tell her that mine were getting pretty leathery, too. She was both intrigued and somewhat knowledgeable about barefoot running, too, having looked up some things herself. Now, perhaps, she will be inspired to give it a try.

The wandering husband/coach showed up around mile 8 with ... jelly beans. He had apparently gone shopping while I had been running. He wanted to make sure I had enough energy *(not being convinced that my 4 cups of lemonade were enough)* and offered me my choice of marshmallow or tangerine jelly beans. I said I would try a few of the tangerine flavored ones. *(Marshmallow sounded horrible and I blocked the thought of them from my mind immediately.)* We passed sandals and plastic bags of jelly beans back and forth so that I could take what I wanted from the bag. I threw about 4 in my mouth, like a good girl. I found I *could* breath through my mouth without choking while chewing jelly beans, and thanked him for taking care of me. Then, he disappeared again while I headed for a pleasant, shaded, riverside greenbelt section of the course.

Why Does Grandma Run Barefoot?

Meeting a woman who was running her 93rd marathon was another highlight of this section of the run. There were so many fun details she was willing to share, while still asking me in a friendly way about my life and running. Her husband was an Olympic marathoner in the 1980's. She has run a marathon in all 50 states. She began running marathons in the 1990's, but took a long break and started up again in 2005. The closest in time she has ever run 2 marathons is on a Thursday, then a Sunday. And, yes, she has run the New York and Boston marathons, however doesn't really recommend them. She likes the smaller races. After she completes 100 marathons, she plans on tackling a 50 K. And she is a few years older than me! She said the last few miles are still always hard for her, but I didn't really get an idea of her training or how frequently she usually runs them. Overall, very fun and encouraging conversation, and memory of it helped me during the last few miles.

The marathon course was the same as the half marathon course for the first 12 and the last 1.2 miles. I mention this particularly because that first half of the course was very easy to run barefoot, especially for someone who has run mostly barefoot for a couple of years. I did utilize some sidewalks, but most of the pavement was smooth to moderate. I was easily able to keep a running pace limited by my aerobic training rather than accommodating rough running surfaces. Thus, if someone is looking for a "barefoot friendly" half marathon, I would recommend this race.

All was still comfortable running until we came to some neighborhood streets in the north end of Boise, near Camel's Back Park. Here, about mile 15, there were not sidewalks and the asphalt was very sharp chip seal. I slipped on my Lunas, as I could not tell how long it would go on and I didn't want the frustration at that point in the race. When sidewalks did show up again, they were uneven and strewn with nuts and leaves, but I knew I wanted to take my sandals off. I was right. Being barefoot felt better. I could cross the rough streets easily enough, as long as I didn't have to run on them constantly. Maybe some day I will be up to that.

During this barefoot time, a tall, fit enough looking man came up puffing beside me. He was intent on telling me that when he began to feel sorry for himself about his legs hurting so much, he just thought about me, running along holding my flip-flops in my hand. The first thing I told him, while I held them up for exhibit, was that they were running sandals! Then, I am afraid I may have discouraged him when I said, *"My feet are happy being bare!"*, shortly thereafter pulling away from him with no effort.

Then I came to another portion of the course in down town Boise that was rough and around a lot of traffic. It was the only part of the course that had cones on both sides of us while we pretty much ran down the middle of busy streets with cars all around us. There were very conscientious volunteers helping to guard our crossings at intersections, but I still felt on high alert, kind of like a scared rabbit. Thus, I was thankful to have my Lunas for that part. We ran past a politically active enclave of homeless people under a bridge, that I was less than receptive to, as they wanted "free housing not free handouts." I was thinking if they put as much effort into job hunting as they were their picketing, they could probably afford housing. Whatever my economic convictions, I was glad there was a manly looking volunteer there, because the homeless folks were looking confrontational and I was feeling vulnerable after 17 miles of running.

I was beginning to get tired now. I took off my sandals again because I had a sense it would make me feel more alive in my running. I was right. Minimalist footwear is better than those toe confining, inflexible footboxes that most people call shoes, but nothing is as good as barefoot in most normal situations.

I still wasn't breathing hard, except for barely at the top of a couple of significant hills. My MAF training was really helping with that. In fact, on that hill, I unintentionally "lost" a few people who had been generally close to me throughout much of the race. One of them was a race walker, who I was trying not to let drive me crazy. It wasn't that she was obnoxious, but her slowing to a walk, then pulling ahead running was not a rhythm that I could adjust to. I was happy that the hill finally separated us.

Why Does Grandma Run Barefoot?

My legs now began getting more leaden with each step. Definitely a case of "so close, yet so far away." I hit some comparatively rough pavement, but surprised myself by realizing that being barefoot now was more of a boost to my energy than rough pavement was an impediment. My pace was already down to what it normally is on rougher pavement, so it was oddly comfortable. I passed about 3 other dogged racers even.

Soon, I hit a down hill that tested my legs in a whole new way. The downhills earlier in the race had been fun, as I glided carefully down them. This time, my legs hurt intensely with every step. I tried not to tense up, so as to cause myself damage. When I got to the bottom, I could not remember the last time I had seen a painted arrow on the road. There hadn't been any volunteers for a couple of miles and I couldn't see any racers in front of me. Fortunately, it had occurred to me to study the race course the day before, and generally being familiar with downtown Boise, it was not hard to bring to mind that I should be at least in the right vicinity. I figured I should run a bit more and was relieved to finally see another arrow pointing to a turn into Ann Morrison Park. I guess that is one drawback of small races. You can end up by yourself at some point.

Come to find out, my husband/coach had been looking for me around there. Seeing how deserted the area was, and knowing my lack of directional ability, he was not sure how or where to look for me. At the same time, he was able to help 2-3 other runners who had accidentally passed the arrows that I had seen. He is so good at keeping track of things, he knew who was ahead and behind me the whole time, so he figured out that he should just go to the finish since he couldn't see me up or down the road and the rest of the course was again on the greenbelt.

Through the circuitous section in Ann Morrison Park, I mostly ran on the pass-through roads. There was one part where I risked running on the grass, whatever hidden objects there might be, because the road was rough, but I knew where the end of it was. I could feel the turf absorbing my bounce, though, and was ironically glad for the paved greenbelt. There were volunteers sitting at that spot, which I was glad of, because I was feeling my mental powers fading and I really wanted some assurance about where to go. I don't think they got nearly as many smiles as the volunteers in the first two-thirds of the course...

One of my biggest concerns about the last few miles was that they would seem sooo long. I am still puzzling over how they seemed to slip by in spite of the slow pace and aching legs. Partly, I think it helped that I didn't spend a lot of time focusing on exactly how far I had to go, but rather mostly thought about putting one foot in front of the other and just making it to the end. That said, I have complete compassion on anyone who gets to that point in the race and feels they cannot make it another step, even with only a mile to go. It hurt. I reminded myself that I had gone through 7 labors without pain relieving drugs, so this was nothing. Okay, not nothing, but doable. Hopefully.

As you may have suspected, I did make it. I even slightly picked up the pace for the last quarter mile. I had to do my best not to be passed so close to the finish line, although I had no clue how close anyone was. Nothing heroic or that could lead to a pulled muscle, not that I was capable of that. I was so pleased to see several of my kids and all my grandkids at the finish area, cheering me on! Then, my 2 year old grandson, unbeknownst to me, started trying to sprint down the chute behind me as fast as his little legs could carry him. I wish I had noticed and could have taken him across with me.

When I was done, I was, um, wobbly. I needed to sit down, but my kids were afraid I wouldn't make it up again. My legs felt they might seize up if I required anything more of them. I made it to a sunny patch of grass with some help. One of them ran to get orange slices for me.

After the race, my 93rd marathoner friend came up to congratulate me. She had finished some seconds behind me. Later, as I made my way past the finish, to our car, another gentleman who was just finishing made it a point to yell over to me that I had run well. I got the impression he was truly astonished that I had done as well as I had with bare feet. A

Why Does Grandma Run Barefoot?

spectator, a woman who was approximately my age and was cheering people in along the finish chute, came over to hug me and tell me what an inspiration I was!

It wasn't that my results were spectacular. All I had wanted to do was finish and have fun.

- It took me 4 hours 50 minutes and 41 seconds to do that, not counting the measly 18 seconds it took to get up to the starting line.
- My pace was an 11:06 average, being closer to a 10 minute mile pace in the first half and closer to a 12 minute mile pace in the second half. It looks like I actually beat my fastest half marathon pace for that distance and that part felt easy!
- I placed 105th overall out of 147 marathoners. (winner's time was 2:32:08)
- 4th in my age group of 8 women 50-59 (the fastest in my age group was 4:09:48)
- 36th out of 66 women total (fastest woman clocked 3:10:40 at age 26)

But it's not about my results. Not for you. It is about where *you* are starting from for your own goals and accomplishments. I completed a marathon, and strange as it ay sound, I am already thinking about preparing for another. It was fun training, the race was exciting, and I am thrilled with my barefooting progress. However, I didn't start with a marathon. I started with getting ready for a 5K. After years of struggling to fit in 20 minutes of exercise only 3 times a week while (happily) raising multiple children. After injuries and surgeries and slow recoveries. After beginning to feel old, then deciding that didn't mean I needed to act old. And I still think I can go faster. Catch me if you can!

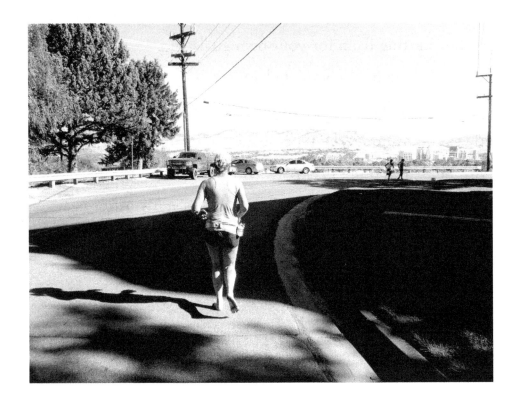

Why Does Grandma Run Barefoot?

Chapter Nine

Barefoot for Life

I didn't set out to be a barefoot grandma, but I am very happy it has worked out that way! I appreciate the people and businesses who don't make a big deal out of me choosing the normal use of my feet. I also am grateful for the people who are willing to have rational conversations about it and reconsider their biases.

For those who are stubborn or trapped in their misconceptions about health or acceptable footwear, I will have to choose my battles, so-to-speak. I'm not trying to be belligerent, but there are very good reasons to be barefoot most of the time. There are times when I will decide to share about being barefoot and why it should be a very rare thing indeed to require shoes on anyone's property.

Meanwhile, if you see me or any other barefoot runner out there, realize we are not doing it to be a spectacle or just be weird. We think it is more normal than wearing shoes. We wish everyone could be as comfortable and having as much fun as we are!

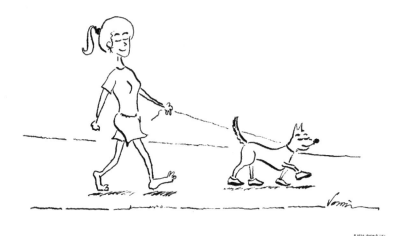

Stay in touch and learn more about being barefoot

To learn more about being barefoot and to follow along in my barefoot fitness activities, please visit funfitnessafter50.com.

I am also barefoot in the garden at dailyimprovisations.com.

<u>Other sources for general barefoot living are:</u>

The Society for Barefoot Living
http://www.barefooters.org

The Barefoot Book, by Daniel Howell, PhD
http://www.thebarefootbook.com/index.html

<u>Recommended books about running barefoot:</u>

Barefoot Running Step by Step, by Roy M. Wallack and
Barefoot Ken Bob Saxton

The Barefoot Running Book: The Art and Science of Barefoot and Minimalist Shoe Running, by Jason Robillard

Barefoot Running by Michael Sandler and Jessica Lee

The Zen of Running by Fred Rohe

Other books by Laura Blodgett:

Melody's Life Savings (the story of one young teenage daughter's experience with leukemia and the legacy she left behind)

The Blue Fish (a children's book)

The Blue Fish in Chinese (a Fun Learning Chinese book)

A Million Rocks - A book of almost counting words (a children's book) (Chinese version coming soon!)

How to Build a Backyard Brick Oven From Scratch , also by Greg Blodgett (a how he did it and you can too book)